THE CANCER MICROBE

D1569303

ALSO BY
ALAN CANTWELL JR.

AIDS: THE MYSTERY AND THE SOLUTION

AIDS AND THE DOCTORS OF DEATH

THE CANCER MICROBE

ALAN CANTWELL JR., M.D.

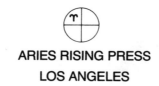

ARIES RISING PRESS
LOS ANGELES

Aries Rising Press
P.O. Box 29532
Los Angeles, CA 90029

The quotations in Chapter 10 from *Every Second Child* (© 1981 by Archie Kalokerinos and Keats Publishing Co, New Canaan, CT) are used with permission.

Library of Congress Cataloging-in-Publication Data

Cantwell, Alan, 1934-
   The cancer microbe / Alan Cantwell, Jr.
      p.   cm.
   Includes bibliographical references.
   ISBN 0-917211-01-4 (soft): $18.95
   1. Cancer—Microbiology—Research—History. 2. Cantwell, Alan,
1934-   . 3. Dermatologists—California—Biography. I. Cantwell,
Alan, 1934-   . II. Title.
   [DNLM: 1. Neoplasms—microbiology—personal narratives.
QZ 201 C234c]
RC262.C295   1990
616.99'401—dc20
DNLM/DLC   90-358
for Library of Congress   CIP

ISBN 0-917211-01-4

Printed in the United States of America

10 9 8 7 6 5 4 3 2 1

Dedicated with love to the memory of my parents,

Alan Ralph Cantwell, M.D., F.A.C.S.
(February 27, 1903 — February 12, 1973)

and

Frances Louise Danforth Cantwell, R.N.
(July 24, 1908 — July 8, 1979)

Whose devotion to the highest ideals of the medical
profession has inspired my quest for the truth

"When science cannot be questioned, it is not science anymore: it is religion."

— Tony Brown
(Tony Brown's Journal)

"There are not different kinds of life, for life is like the truth. It does not have degrees. It is the one condition in which all that God created share. Like all His Thoughts, it has no opposite. There is no death because what God created shares His Life. There is no death because an opposite to God does not exist. There is no death because the Father and the Son are one."

— A Course in Miracles

TABLE OF CONTENTS

Chapter 1   The Forgotten Microbe   11
Chapter 2   The Young Physician   17
Chapter 3   The Dermatologist   33
Chapter 4   Reuben's Scleroderma   43
Chapter 5   Livingston's *Progenitor cryptocides* . . .   53
Chapter 6   Alexander-Jackson and Pleomorphism   71
Chapter 7   The Sarcoidosis Connection   85
Chapter 8   The Cancer Microbe   103
Chapter 9   Bechamp's Microzymas   121
Chapter 10   Bechamp or Pasteur?   141
Chapter 11   Reich's Bions   155
Chapter 12   Reich's Orgone Energy   175
Chapter 13   AIDS and Biological Warfare   185
Chapter 14   The Old Physician   221
Microphotographs   232
Subject Index   273
Index of Proper Names   277
About the Author   283

ACKNOWLEDGEMENTS

THE CANCER MICROBE reflects my life and my career as a physician-scientist. Many outstanding research scientists are included in this book, and I am indebted to each of them for their contributions to the field of cancer microbiology.

A special thanks goes to my microbiologist friends: Eugenia Craggs, Dan Kelso, Joyce E. Jones, and Lida Mattman, Ph.D., for their efforts in instructing me in the art and science of bacteriology. The very special knowledge contained in Professor Lida Mattman's remarkable book, *CELL WALL DEFICIENT FORMS,* has been a constant source of inspiration in my investigation into the bacteriology of cancer.

My cancer microbe research could never have been undertaken without the aid of four women scientists who are pioneers in the microbiology of cancer: Virginia Livingston M.D., Eleanor Alexander-Jackson, Ph.D., Florence Seibert, Ph.D., and the late Irene Diller, Ph.D. I am deeply honored to have known them all.

My concept of AIDS as biowarfare derives from my association with Robert Strecker, M.D., one of the most brilliant and courageous physicians I have ever known. I thank Glen Dettman, Ph.D., and Dorothy Knafelc for their contributions to my study of Antoine Bechamp, and I appreciate their willingness to allow me to quote from their letters and writings.

For the story of Wilhelm Reich I was profoundly influenced by David Boadella's *WILHELM REICH: THE EVOLUTION OF HIS WORK* (Vision Press, Chicago); Myron Sharaf's *FURY ON EARTH* (St. Martin's Press, New York); and by Reich's *THE CANCER BIOPATHY* and *THE BION EXPERIMENTS,* both published by Farrar, Straus, and Giroux, New York.

To my editor, Suzanne Henig, Ph. D., I extend my thanks and appreciation for her efforts in finalizing the manuscript for publication.

A special thank-you goes to Helvi Lansu, and to my partner, Frank A. Sinatra, who is always there for me.

Last, but not least, I am indebted to my research patients who have taught me about the cancer microbe, its significance, and its origin.

CHAPTER ONE

The Forgotten Microbe

As a young boy back in the 1940s, I remember reading about the great scientists of the last century who revolutionized medicine by discovering microbes. The most famous was Louis Pasteur, the French chemist who proved that microbes could cause human disease. Within a few years the microbes that caused tuberculosis, syphilis and leprosy were discovered. These biomedical breakthroughs ushered in the golden age of twentieth century modern medicine.

Later, as a young physician I assumed that all the bacterial microbes which caused serious diseases had been discovered. I never dreamed I would encounter the most remarkable and the most important germ of all — the microbe of cancer.

Forgotten and ignored in the medical libraries of the world is a wealth of scientific knowledge on the cancer microbe. My awareness of this knowledge has given greater meaning to my life as a medical doctor and as a scientific researcher. It is now time to share my experiences with the cancer microbe with those who are seeking a better understanding of cancer.

Although it has been recognized for a century, the cancer microbe still remains unknown to most physicians and cancer scientists because knowledge of its existence is not transmitted through medical school courses anywhere in the world. This is unfortunate because the cancer microbe plays a vitally important role in the development of cancer.

For the past three decades I have observed and studied the cancer microbe. It can be easily seen by using a standard microscope of the type available in medical laboratories and doctor's offices.

It is difficult for doctors to conceive of a cancer microbe because one of the first things a medical student learns is that cancer is not a contagious or infectious disease. Doctors are taught that bacteria can be detected microscopically in diseases like TB, leprosy, and syphilis. But medical professors teach that no bacteria can be detected in cancer. Therefore, the idea of a bacterial microbe in cancer is considered unscientific, and unworthy of investigation and comment.

Most doctors scoff at the idea of a cancer microbe. Scientists occasionally concede that bacteria can be found in cancer, but they claim that such bacteria are "contaminants" or "secondary invaders" which invade the weakened tissue after the cancer is formed. Physicians insist that such bacteria have nothing to do with the actual "cause" of cancer.

Currently, many physicians believe that certain forms of cancer may be caused by viruses, such as the newly-discovered AIDS virus. Viruses differ from bacteria in certain ways. Bacteria can survive and grow outside the cell, but viruses can live only within the cell. Another difference is that bacteria can be visualized microscopically, but viruses are too small to be seen with a standard microscope. Viruses can be visualized only with an electron microscope which magnifies up to 100,000 times or more.

Despite the medical profession's rejection of bacteria in cancer, there are many researchers who have studied various aspects of the cancer microbe. In most instances, their reports have appeared in highly specialized scientific journals. Some reports have been published in foreign journals, particularly in Germany and France. Other scientific papers exist in journals which are now defunct. As a result, most of the century-old information on cancer bacteria lies buried in the scientific literature, unlikely to be retrieved except by the most dedicated and open-minded cancer researchers who know where to look and who are fluent in German and French.

Like Louis Pasteur and other well-known microbiologists of the last century, I am a microbe hunter and my prey is the microbe of cancer. The cancer microbe is easy to detect. The published reports explain how cancer bacteria can be detected in cancerous tissue, and how cancer microbes can be grown in the laboratory. Cancer bacteria are as easy to demonstrate as the bacteria that cause TB, leprosy, and syphilis.

Most of my colleagues ignore my published cancer microbe research because they are convinced that cancer microbes do not exist. A few sympathetic physicians have suggested that I become a full-time cancer researcher and verse myself in all the latest biotechnology in order to prove, beyond doubt, that bacteria exist in cancer. They recommend that I apply for a government grant, acquire a team of expert laboratory workers, and align myself with a prestigious medical university which could oversee and direct my research.

I have often mused about these suggestions, but they are out of touch with my talents and training. The idea of becoming a full-time researcher to prove what I already know seems foolish, particularly when there is already adequate scientific evidence to prove that the cancer microbe exists.

All controversial researchers are plagued by self-doubts about the validity and worth of their work. Because my cancer discoveries seriously conflict with estabished scientific dogma, I have often experienced fear, depression, anger, uncertainty, and professional isolation. And yet, my belief in the cancer microbe is so strong that I have persisted in studying it for more than 25 years. I cannot dismiss the microbe as a figment of my imagination. Too many scientists whose work I respect have reported similar observations. Too many have been denied official recognition, and have been targets of investigation by official governmental bodies determined to shut down their medical and research practices.

Because of my unorthodox beliefs I have become a medical revolutionary and an idealist disillusioned with the "science" of medicine. In truth, I have learned there is no such thing as medical science; there are only scientists whose collective knowledge becomes what is accepted and known as medical science.

In reality, medicine is more an art than a science. So-called medical science may prove to be yet another worldly illusion, albeit a potent and necessary one. For example, twentieth century medical science is totally unlike medical science of the last century. Medical historians can attest to the fact that nineteenth century scientists were a somewhat foolish and ignorant group of men who blamed all diseases on the ethers, the miasms of the air, the work of the devil, or the wrath of God. Throughout most of the last century, most medical doctors were totally unaware that microbes could cause human disease! The few physicians who tried to alert their colleagues to the possible dangers of infectious microbes were called heretics, or worse.

As I begin my story, I trust that I will be able to relate my knowledge of the cancer microbe in a way that is simple to understand for readers who have no training in biomedical subjects. For those medically-trained professionals who seek "peer-reviewed" publications on the subject, I offer my technical writings on the microbiology of cancer, which are available in medical libraries throughout the world.

It is disconcerting that the leaders in medical science have chosen to disregard cancer microbe research. Nevertheless, I believe the public should be made aware of the existence and the importance of the cancer microbe. Their lives potentially depend on this knowledge. For this reason I will attempt to explain, in simple terms, the microbiologic principles necessary to understand the germ of cancer.

In the process of explaining my scientific experiences with the cancer microbe, I feel compelled to relate some personal life experiences which have greatly influenced my cancer research. It is ordinarily considered inappropriate for scientists to mix personal life into biomedical research. However, I know no other way to explain the driving forces that led me into cancer research, and ultimately into AIDS research. In short, my scientific work has always been so intertwined with my personal life, that I can no longer meaningfully explain the one without the other.

The cancer germ staggers the mind. The microbe lives within us, and is an integral part of every living cell in our body. But the cancer microbe is much more than a microbe of death. The cancer microbe is also intimately connected with healing and with the "life force." Within the cells of all living creatures is contained an energy

force of intense magnitude that permeates our physical
realm. One day we will learn to harness this life force
and we will use it to heal cancer and other diseases of
man! But this cannot happen unless we recognize its
existence.

But I must start at the beginning. And I will tell you
what I have learned in my search for the cancer
microbe. . .

And in the search for my own identity and origin.

CHAPTER TWO

The Young Physician

From the very beginning it was planned that I would be a physician; and my path to medical school was made easier by the fact that Father was a doctor, and Mother a nurse.

Shortly before my birth my Father, Angelo Raphael Cantelmo, legally changed his name to Alan Ralph Cantwell. His Italian family was furious and blamed his red-haired, freckled-faced, social-climbing, Anglo wife. They said he should have married one of his own kind. But, in truth, Father bitterly resented being called "guinea" and "wop" and he didn't want his kids to deal with that kind of prejudice. Three children were born: Alan Ralph, Howard Danforth, and Frances Louise. And they all had American names. As the firstborn I was named after Father. Dad wanted me to be a physician, and Mother agreed wholeheartedly.

My first doll was Doctor Dafoe. Over and over again, Mother told me that Doctor Dafoe was the baby-doctor from Canada who took care of the Dionne quintuplets in a hospital that was built especially for them. I was born on January 4, 1934; the five Dionne girls were born in June of that year. They were the most famous babies in the world and Allan Roy Dafoe was the best doctor. Someday I would grow up and wear a white uniform and carry a stethoscope around my neck, just like Doctor Dafoe.

Five decades later I read a book about Doctor Dafoe and how he and the Canadian government conspired to take the quints away from their parents. The children were housed in a specially-built government hospital that, during the late 1930s and the 1940s, became both the most popular Canadian tourist attraction and the quints' prison. The sordid account in John Nihmey and Stuart Foxman's book, *TIME OF THEIR LIVES: THE DIONNE TRAGEDY* (1986), made me shudder; and it destroyed my first illusion about the best doctor in the whole world.

As far back as I can remember, Mother would ask, "What are you going to be when you grow up?" And I was taught to answer, "A doctor! A doctor like Doctor Dafoe." Mother told everyone I was going to be a physician and "follow in my father's footsteps." There was never any question about that. There were brief moments when I imagined a life as a piano player, or even a dancer. But I knew that would break my parents' hearts, and I would never risk losing their love.

I was the proverbial good boy, attending Catholic school and never missing Sunday mass; the bright and diligent student who breezed his way through high school and into the Ivy League College of his choice. At Cornell University I was immediately submerged in the fierce competitiveness of the pre-med students. I was seventeen and intent on proving my popularity and brilliance. My parents had always told me I was special; now I had to prove it. But it was unbelievably difficult. Compared to the handsome, athletic hunks that attracted the best-looking girls on campus, I was a mess. My face was full of acne, my hair was balding at an alarming rate, and my body urgently needed a crash course in bodybuilding. By the end of the first college semester I was placed on probation for poor grades, and I received the ultimate social rejection by not receiving a bid to join a fraternity. My world had fallen apart and I was crushed.

Father insisted on a conference with the Dean of Cornell. Dad was a fighter who had struggled against all odds to become a physician. During the Depression, he was a family doctor in a poor neighborhood in the Bronx, but he wasn't fully satisfied. He wanted to be an orthopedic surgeon. In 1942, he passed his specialty examinations, and opened his orthopedic practice on Park Avenue in Manhattan. His greatest love was teaching and he was quickly appointed Associate Professor of Orthopedics at New York Medical College. His dream was eventually to give up his private practice and to become Full Professor of Orthopedics at the College.

Dad told the Dean that it was imperative that I get good grades in order to be accepted into medical school. The Dean reassured him that he would do his best to ensure it. I deeply resented Dad's meddling, but I "buckled down" as he demanded, and my grades improved dramatically.

I soon realized I was not an outstanding science student. I detested cutting up frogs and cats in anatomy class, and I hated the stench of the laboratory. I knew that if I were to stand any chance at all of getting into medical school, I would have to drop my major in science and concentrate on courses like history and literature, which I much preferred. I carefully explained all this to Father, who was forced to agree. My strategy worked. My excellent grades in these subjects pulled up my average grades in the required science courses.

By senior year, Dad assured me he could get me into medical school if I could prove to the Admissions Committee that I could get an outstanding grade in quantitative chemistry — one of the toughest bioscience courses at Cornell. I gave up all social activity and concentrated solely on study. I had to prove I was medical school "material." Miraculously, I succeeded. I received one of the top grades awarded that year in chemistry.

The Admissions Committee was impressed and I was accepted into New York Medical College. I knew I would never have been accepted without my father's faculty connections because all my other med school applications were rejected.

I had gone through a four-year trial of fire only to start over again. This time the new four-year test would be much harder. This time my classmates were all the best and the brightest.

Thus began a period of intense loneliness and isolation. I was twenty-one and despite cosmetic facial surgery for acne scarring I was still plagued with zits. I was so neurotic about my bald head that I purchased a wig and lived in fear that my secret would be discovered. Never finding time or energy to exercise, my body was puny; and I was probably the only male virgin in my class.

I commuted three hours daily from my parents' house to medical school in Manhattan. After classes I hurried home to an early dinner, followed by three or four hours of intense study. I had never studied so hard in my life, but it was still not enough. At the end of the first semester, I was placed on probation. Dad and I were devastated. I would have to study harder, especially on weekends. I simply could not fail after having come this far.

I managed to do better, constantly fighting the

nagging fear that I would never become a doctor. Even now, I have terrifying nightmares of medical school. I am scheduled to take an examination that I must pass to graduate, but for some inexplicable reason I have not studied and I am unprepared. I stare at the test paper, but I can't comprehend the questions. My classmates are all writing answers on their exam papers. I cannot pass the test; I know nothing. I will fail. My heart is pounding furiously and I can't breathe. Mercifully, I awaken drenched in perspiration. I thank God it is only that damned recurring nightmare. I'm OK. I have graduated from medical school. I am a doctor. I am safe.

With my youth spent in study and preparation, I still look upon the first half of my life with sadness. My friends were marrying and having kids. But for me, love did not exist. My life was medicine, and it absorbed all my energy.

My last year of medical school was a series of ugly images I can still recall vividly. The worst were the death pronouncements on ambulance duty: a young white man slumped over the back seat of a car on a bitterly cold winter's night on an abandoned street in Harlem. A gunshot through his head; another drug deal gone sour. . .

A black infant, a crib death in a dimly lit, filthy apartment in a decaying Harlem tenement. The horror of trying unsuccessfully to find a place to write my medical report amidst the maddening swarms of roaches covering the walls, the floors, and the furniture.

Even the last few days before graduation were depressing. I was called on a lazy Sunday afternoon to examine a barely conscious black woman who had been admitted to the medical ward. According to the chart she was forty-four, but looked years older. I forced open her eyelids and noted the yellow, jaundiced eyes. Her arms and legs were emaciated, and the abdomen bloated. The skin was dry, the hair scraggly and thin, the fingernails strangely painted with dark blue nail polish. From time to time, her eyes faintly opened and she gazed at me with a weariness that characterizes someone burned out on life.

She desperately needed intravenous fluids but her veins were useless after years of drug abuse. I requested a surgical kit and deadened her wrist with an anesthetic. As I began to cut into her skin to find a suitable vein for the life-saving fluids she required, a black orderly entered the room and came to her bedside. He was silent for a moment, looking at her and then at me. Finally he asked, "Do you know who this is?"

What a strange question! The chart said Eleanora McKay. What was he talking about?

"This is Billie Holiday," he said flatly.

My hands quivered as I studied her face more intently. There was a vague resemblance to the drawing of a face I remembered on one of her albums in my record collection. I gently let go of her wrist and put the scalpel aside. I phoned the Chief Resident, a foreign doctor from Turkey, and told him to come quickly. A celebrity at Metropolitan General Hospital was a rarity and the hospital brass and the reporters would soon be hovering around Billie Holiday's deathbed. I was still a student practicing medicine without a degree, and I wanted the resident to be there to answer their questions.

Poor Billie. I had never heard anyone sing with such feeling, passion, and despair. Over the next few weeks she rallied a bit and even made the headlines when a nurse noticed "treacherous flakes of white powder on Billie's nose" and "a silver-foil package of powder clutched in her hand." The headlines read: "BILLIE CAUGHT WITH HEROIN IN HOSPITAL." She died shortly thereafter. It was a sad ending to my year at Metropolitan.

Our graduation ceremony was marked by violence. Striking hospital workers on picket lines clashed with our class procession as we marched down Fifth Avenue to commencement services at the New York Academy of Medicine. Some classmates, all dressed in cap and gown, were pictured on the cover of the *New York Daily News* (June 10, 1959) with the headline: "STRIKERS RIOT, SHAKE NEW MD'S. STORM GRADUATION; 7 ARRESTED."

I had to get far away from my family, and from the madness and violence of New York. I chose an internship at Mercy Hospital in San Diego. My parents and my brother and sister accompanied me to the airport. There were tearful goodbyes.

Arriving at Los Angeles airport, I went into the men's room and entered a cubicle. Taking the adhesive remover from my shaving kit, I removed my toupee for the last time. It was summer in Southern California and I was finally free to begin my new life, far from the struggles of medical school and the protective influence of my parents. I yearned to surf in the Pacific and feel the pounding of the waves against my body; and I didn't want to be bothered with that damn wig ever again. I was sick of gluing on hair. I had finally made peace with my bald head and threw the toupee in the trash.

The bus to San Diego soon passed the parapets of Disneyland. As it travelled south through the colorful beach towns of Capistrano and Oceanside, I caught glimpses of the ocean as it sparkled in the late afternoon sun. Off in the distance I could spot the silhouettes of small figures on surfboards awaiting the next perfect wave. The trip to San Diego was magical. I knew I could never go back to New York. California was now home.

At Mercy Hospital we were a group of seven interns. I had my own room and we could eat anything we wanted at no charge in the hospital coffee shop. For companionship, I joined a singles Catholic group. There were excursions to nearby Tijuana and the bullfights, and trips north to Big Sur and San Francisco. It was a wonderful year.

At Christmastime I invited my girlfriend Jan from New York to visit. We had dated off and on for several years and I promised to show her Southern California. Jan was bright, attractive, Italian and Catholic; and she was crazy about me. Her parents assumed we would marry, and allowed her to vacation with me.

On the surface it was simple being Catholic. Sex outside of marriage was taboo and I took my religion seriously. Jan came to California secretly expecting to become engaged. Consequently, she was willing to go much further in lovemaking than ever before, trusting that we would never go "all the way." I was smart enough to know that deflowering a virtuous Italian was a serious prelude to marriage.

I will always be grateful to Jan for her tenderness, and for making me realize that I simply was not capable of loving her, or any other woman. As we kissed and explored each other as we had never done before, she teemed with sexuality. But I could no longer fool myself. There was something drastically wrong with my sexual feelings. I knew marriage would be a disaster for both of us.

Perhaps I was a good actor, or maybe she was more deeply in love with me than I could ever imagine, but she never questioned my ardor. After she returned home, I wrote explaining as gently as I could that I did not love her enough to marry her. I tried to make her understand that I would be a poor choice for a husband. She telephoned, heartbroken. She cried and pleaded for me to reconsider. Finally, in desperation she accused me of taking advantage of her. How could I have done those things if I had no intention of marrying her? She cursed me for ruining her life. A year later she married an Italian man and, as far as I know, she was a virgin on her wedding night.

I could hardly have told Jan that I was gay. I still was not exactly sure myself. My first homosexual experience was two years earlier, with a medical school classmate. I was 23 years old. I had always thought I was devoid of sexual feeling — a freak of nature. The first time I made love I was catapaulted to the heights of sexual bliss. Seconds after the act was over, I was revulsed with shame. In 1957, being "queer" was a perversion of the worst order and a definite sign of mental illness. Not only could I rot in hell, but I could be forced into electric shock treatment by psychiatrists, and even institutionalized for homosexuality.

I secretly lived with my guilt, blocking out my sexual emotions and hating my friend for what we did together. A year later we resumed our intense sexual relationship. He eventually married and raised a large family. He still considers himself gay, but is committed to his lifelong relationship with his wife.

At age 25, after my breakup with Jan, I slowly

entered the homosexual world. Matt, one of the interns, sensed that I was gay and invited me to the homosexual bars in San Diego. A new world opened up that I never dreamed existed.

Matt was patient and understood my excitement, as well as my fears concerning my sexual identity. He was my first gay friend and I admired how easily he reveled in his sexual lifestyle. I had thought that all homosexuals were psychiatrically disturbed in some way, but Matt was definitely a happy homosexual.

A quarter of a century later he consulted me professionally. Matt had the early signs and symptoms of AIDS-related complex, and he had stopped having sex with his lover of twenty years. He still had that air of confidence and sophistication that I envied, and that hearty laugh that made me think he would never succumb to this hideous new disease. But he was doomed. He died of AIDS in 1988.

When my internship ended in the summer of 1960, there was no more time to explore my sexual longings. My year of freedom was over. I received my military orders to report to Fort Sam Houston, in San Antonio, Texas.

When I started college in 1951, the Korean war was raging. College men were deferred from the draft only if they enrolled in the reserved officer's training program. I signed up immediately, reasoning it was a lot better than dying in a rice paddy in Korea. I was trained to be a "forward observer," an officer who scouts in advance of the troops and spots targets for bombing. In the Korean war the mortality rate for forward observers was staggering.

When I graduated from Cornell in 1955 I received my

commission as a Second Lieutenant in the infantry. However, having been accepted into medical school, the Army deferred me until after my internship. Instead of using me as a forward observer, the Army would use me as a doctor.

As an Army Medical Officer I again shut off my sexual emotions. I joined a military world of men trained in the art of killing. And in this world it is considered manly to riddle an enemy with bullets; but it is never OK to touch a man sexually.

After basic training at Fort Sam Houston I was assigned to a unit located a few miles south of the demilitarized zone separating North and South Korea. This was my new home for fifteen lonely months. It seemed that loneliness was a permanent, never-ending part of my life.

When I arrived in Korea in the fall of 1960, the bloody war had ended seven years earlier. My combat unit was part of the United Nations peacekeeping force. Our mission was to repel the North Korean communists in case of a renewed attack against the South. I was the official health-keeper for several thousand young men cooped up in a barren and dusty valley. On that base in Korea I learned more about male sexuality than is ever written in the textbooks. I also discovered some surprising facts about official Army record-keeping.

The Koreans were barely recovering from the disastrous war, and the villages surrounding the military camps were swarming with prostitutes eager to meet the needs of frustrated soldiers. The men wanted sex and the prostitutes desperately needed money. As a result of this classic example of the law of supply and demand, venereal disease (VD) was rampant.

Most of the morning clinic hours were spent treating

dozens of infected men each day. It was rare for a military man to escape VD during his Korean tour of duty. I had naively assumed that the officers, especially the married ones, would have some control over their sexual passions. The officers constantly lectured about military discipline and morality, and repeatedly chastised the enlisted men for the alarming VD rates in the unit.

Many officers came to me for private treatment of sexually-transmitted diseases. My staff-sergeant goodnaturedly but sternly advised me never to record an officer's VD infection in the medical record. Thus, I quickly learned why VD was practically non-existent among the officers. Since my military days I have always looked askance at government statistics. They are often padded to produce the "result" the government wants to portray. This is particularly true of the current AIDS epidemic statistics.

It was impossible for any man (straight or gay) to avoid the Korean prostitutes. Many were beautiful and surprisingly unrestrained in their sexuality. To break the monotony at the base, I occasionally travelled to Seoul with some married officers I had befriended. After a few drinks at the cocktail lounge, they quickly forgot their wives back home and began to make sexual arrangements with the bargirls. Getting laid in Seoul was as easy as snapping your fingers. Within minutes there was a girl for each of us, and soon we were all romping assnaked in our hotel room.

There was really no way to avoid these situations. To the military mind, it would have been unthinkable and unmanly to decline the heterosexual pleasures that were cheap and plentiful in Korea in the 1960s. The so-called sexual revolution in America in the 1970s was hardly noticeable to military men who had served in Asia.

Although most servicemen were anxious to leave Korea, the sexual lure proved so addicting that some men sheepishly signed up for an additional tour of duty. For those men, the good life was the erotic pleasures of Korea that could never be duplicated back home in the States.

At age 28, I was continuing to suppress my true sexual feelings, knowing full well the taboo of homosexuality in the military. At the same time I was trying to hang on to the last vestiges of my Catholic moralistic upbringing. On our military base where the days were focused on war and the nights were focused on sex, Christian principles seemed hopelessly outdated.

One of the few benefits of Korea was that I had plenty of time to think about what I wanted to do with my life. I decided on dermatology and I applied to every residency program in California, and to a program in New York. I also requested reassignment to Fort MacArthur Army Hospital in Los Angeles. Luckily, my military application was approved.

I left Korea in January 1962, infinitely wiser in the ways of the world. Before starting my new tour of duty, I visited the family in New York.

Father was feeling poorly, and Mother was worried. He was showing the first symptoms of a neurologic disease which would soon destroy his life. Mother confided that his illness started shortly after his dream for full professorship at the medical college was shattered.

During my absence in Korea, Mother and Dad attended a big formal gala at the college. After dinner the faculty big-wigs began their speeches at the dais. The Professor of Orthopedics rose to give a surprise announcement. Dad was curious about what his superior would say. The Professor was delighted to announce that, after careful deliberation, he had chosen a new head for the orthopedic department, The new professor had fabulous credentials and the college was indeed fortunate to have coaxed him away from the finest medical school in Philadelphia.

At first, it was difficult for Father to comprehend what his superior was saying. Dad was next in line for professorship and for many years he had worked tirelessly teaching orthopedics to the residents and the med students. All the doctors loved him. He never received a penny for his time and effort; it was just assumed that he would be chosen to head the department when the current professor retired. That was the way staff physicians were usually repaid for years of free service to the medical school.

The announcement stunned Father. The energy drained from his body and he felt like he was going to die. He had to get out of the ballroom. Trembling, he slowly rose from the dinner table while his colleagues looked on in silence. He had just received the most crushing disappointment of his career and he was devastated with embarrassment and shame. Mother lovingly put her hand in his, and holding her head proudly, she gently led him out of the room.

He was never the same after that. Little tremors began in his muscles, his speech slurred, and he was unsteady on his feet. The examining neurologists thought it was psychological, but when the symptoms worsened they diagnosed his condition as "amyotrophic lateral sclerosis" (Lou Gehrig's disease), a progressively fatal nerve disease for which there is no treatment and no known cause. Father was still performing surgery, but he feared his hands would fail him. Eventually they did.

There was little I could do to cheer up my parents, but I did have some good news. Although all my applications to dermatology programs in California were rejected, I was accepted at the nearby Bronx VA Hospital. My training would begin in September 1962, after my military obligation was over.

In the interim I looked forward to six more months in California at Fort MacArthur. The Commanding Officer notified me that I would be functioning as a pediatrician at the base. I brushed up on the subject of children's diseases, aided considerably by a Greek woman pediatrician who had been hired on as a civilian.

The army hospital was minutes away from Hollywood. I contacted my intern friend Matt, who was now practicing in Beverly Hills. He welcomed me back to America and back into the gay life.

The year 1962 changed my life completely. My youth was rapidly fading away and before it was gone I wanted to fall in love. Nineteen sixty-two brought that opportunity. It was the best year of my life — and the worst.

Matt invited me to my first gay party and I was alive with anticipation. I was introduced to a strikingly handsome man and I felt an electrifying attraction unlike anything I had ever experienced. I had never met anyone like Bob. He was friendly, interesting, animated, and totally charming. He invited me to his tiny one-room Hollywood apartment and switched-on his prized Grundig radio, which was magically tuned to a classical music station. When we touched I felt like I was being touched for the first time. I had never experienced such bliss. In that moment my life unalterably changed direction. I was no longer alone and lonely. I was in love for the first time, and after a few weeks I knew I could never leave Bob and go back to New York.

Impulsively I wrote the Bronx VA Hospital, explaining that I had decided to go into practice in Los Angeles. I didn't know how I would make a living, but I knew I could find work as a physician. I wanted to be a dermatologist but there was nothing more important than being with Bob. Nothing.

I was young and in love and I thought it would last forever.

CHAPTER THREE

The Dermatologist

Compared to Korea my tour of duty at Fort MacArthur was a dream. I was amazed at how quickly I was transformed into a "pediatrician." Fortunately, the Army paid civilian specialists to take care of the more complicated cases. Once a week we had a special skin clinic and Meyer Berke, a Long Beach dermatologist, was the civilian consultant at the Fort.

When I told Meyer that I wanted to study dermatology, he suggested that I apply at the nearby Long Beach VA Hospital where he was on staff. I explained that my application had already been rejected there. Meyer still thought I should meet with Professor Becker in person.

Sam Becker was sixty eight years old and well past the normal age of retirement for the VA. However, because of his extraordinary reputation in dermatology the VA kept him on as Professor Emeritus. I found him aloof and unfriendly. He reviewed my rejected application and bluntly reminded me that my grades in medical school were below average. I explained that I wanted to become a dermatologist and asked him to keep me in mind if a position came up in his department. Becker seriously doubted that a vacancy would occur because there were many more applicants than there were positions in his derm residency program.

Six weeks later I received a call to meet with Dr. Becker. At the meeting, Sam explained that a woman was supposed to have started training, but she got pregnant and cancelled. He remarked that he usually didn't hire women because he found them undependable. Now he was obviously annoyed that he had to fill the vacancy at the last minute.

Finally Sam said, "Ordinarily I wouldn't hire someone with your credentials. You are not well qualified. However, if you want the position, I will accept you. Can you start in July?"

I could hardly believe my ears. "Sir, my army discharge date is September 1st. I have to be in my brother's wedding in New York the first week in September. Would the second week in September be all right?"

Sam nodded weakly and dismissed me. I prayed that he would never find out about the derm residency I turned down in New York. He never did.

The six months at Fort MacArthur were over in a flash. Bob and I leased a small Hollywood apartment. It was an hour's drive to Long Beach but I didn't care. I was in love and everything was falling into place. I had never been so lucky.

I returned to New York for my brother's wedding. Howard was now a medical student at New York Medical College and Father was extremely proud of his two doctor sons. It was sad to see Father's rapid deterioration, but he still insisted on dancing a few feeble steps with Mom.

When I returned to Los Angeles, Bob picked me up at the airport. I had missed him terribly and told him so. He was quiet as we drove to Hollywood. When we entered the apartment, I threw my arms around him but he gently pushed me away. "What's wrong?" I asked.

"It's hard for me to tell you. But it's over. I can't love you anymore. I just want to be friends."

"What are you talking about? What did I do?" I couldn't comprehend what was happening. "We just got this apartment. I'm starting a new job in Long Beach. . . and you tell me it's over?"

It was over. I had known Bob for only six short, deliriously happy months. Until Bob, I had never loved anyone and now I didn't know how to stop loving him.

The next few weeks were unbearable, seeing him come and go from the apartment, and waiting for him to come home in the wee hours of the morning. For the first time in my life I seriously considered suicide. I had to get away from Bob and find a place of my own. It was the only way to ease the pain.

Alone and depressed, and without close friends, I started my residency with a heavy heart. As the months passed, I avoided Dr. Becker as much as I could. I sensed there was nothing I could do to please him, and I always seemed to say the wrong thing.

I remember the day President Kennedy was assassinated. A few of us were huddled around the clinic radio, stunned by the news. Sam Becker came by and asked me what was happening.

"Kennedy's been fatally shot," I responded sadly.

"They should have killed that son-of-a-bitch a long time ago," he grumbled as he left the room.

Sam Becker died suddenly the following summer. I will never forget him for taking me on as a resident, but it was hard to grieve his passing.

The only thing I admired about him was his total dedication to dermatology. In one of his lighter moods he confided that his best vacations were spent studying the dermatology literature at the medical library at UCLA. At the time, I thought that was a rather dreary

way to enjoy a holiday. Years later I surprised myself by
taking vacations for the sole purpose of medical research
and writing. Maybe Sam and I were similar, in some
ways. Sometimes I wonder if I got involved in dermatology research just to outshine Sam.

My search for the cancer microbe started quite by
accident, and in a way that I never suspected would
change the entire course of my life. It began in the
medical library at the Long Beach VA Hospital. I had
gathered a pile of dermatology journals around me,
hoping to find something of interest to present at the
weekly Medical Journal Club meeting. Eventually I
came across a curious report describing patients who
developed skin infections after receiving allergy injections.
The reporting doctors discovered that the allergy
medication bottles were contaminated with tuberculosis-
type microbes. The report reminded me of Willa, one of
my patients.
   Willa was a World War II veteran. For years
afterward she suffered from mental problems. She
constantly complained of a maddening itch and painful
lumps deep in the skin of her buttocks. She was often
dirty and unkempt, with a strange look in her eyes that
hinted at her mental instability. But there was also
something fragile about her that made me want to help
her. I painstakingly explained that her itch would
improve during periods when she was less nervous. She
understood perfectly, and this was no big problem for
her. But the bumps on her buttocks were another
matter. They were painful and tender, and it was
uncomfortable for her to sit. Willa often cried when she
talked about her bumps. She complained that none of us
knew what was causing them, or how to make them go

away.

Remembering the report about tuberculosis (TB) infection following injections of medication, I asked Willa if injections might have caused her bumps. She recalled the swellings started four years earlier, when she was hospitalized for convulsions in 1959. The painful lumps started soon after she was given injections of sedatives and antibiotics.

Willa agreed to let me cut out one of the largest and deepest lesions to test for TB bacteria. Part of the skin sample was sent to the histology lab where the tissue was "fixed" with chemicals and embedded into small blocks of paraffin wax. A machine sliced Willa's tissue into paper-thin "sections." The histologic technician carefully placed the tissue sections onto glass slides and stained the tissue with the hematoxylin-eosin stain. After drying, a thin glass cover slip was placed over the material and the slides were sent to the pathologist for examination.

Another piece of Willa's skin tissue was sent to bacteriology for TB culture. Eugenia Craggs, the senior technician in the TB lab, ground-up Willa's tissue and placed a bit of it on a glass slide and colored the tissue with an "acid-fast" stain. The acid-fast stain colors TB germs red; and colors the tissue blue.

When Eugenia examined Willa's stained tissue, she detected typical acid-fast, red-stained, rod-shaped bacteria. Eugenia could not tell exactly what kind of a TB germ it was. She would know after the culture grew and was tested biochemically. Eugenia phoned to tell me that Willa's smear was "positive for TB-type, acid-fast bacteria."

There are many different "species" of acid-fast mycobacteria. For example, *Mycobacterium tuberculo-*

sis causes TB; and *Mycobacterium leprae* causes leprosy. Other species of mycobacteria are called "atypical mycobacteria," and these may (or may not) cause TB and other infections. Some acid-fast mycobacteria are harmless. Unlike most bacteria, TB mycobacteria grow slowly and may take as long as several months to grow in laboratory culture.

Most TB germs prefer to grow at a special temperature on solid laboratory "media" containing special nutritive ingredients. Some species of mycobacteria prefer to grow in a fluid medium. For this reason, Eugenia also planted some of Willa's tissue in a special liquid broth.

Although Eugenia detected acid-fast bacteria in Willa's ground-up tissue, Eugenia could not culture typical acid-fast bacteria. Instead, a microbe which looked like a fungus was cultured. The germ was not acid-fast, and no one in the lab was sure of its exact identity.

Willa's strange-looking fungus was sent to Ruth Gordon, a noted bacteriologist, at the Institute of Microbiology at Rutgers University. After much study, she identified the fungus as *Streptomyces coelicolor.* Nobody in the dermatology department had ever heard of this germ. And it wasn't mentioned in the medical textbooks.

The pathologist observed inflammation deep in the fat portion (the panniculus) of Willa's skin and diagnosed her disease as "panniculitis," but no acid-fast bacteria were found in the tissue sections.

I detected tiny, pink-stained "granules" in Willa's acid-fast stained tissue sections. There were also peculiar-looking, large balloon-like forms deep in Willa's fat tissue. The pathologist ignored the "granules." He wasn't exactly sure what they were but, in his opinion, they were definitely not microbes. He interpreted the bizarre balloon forms as "degeneration" of Willa's fat.

Over a period of months, I excised five more lumps from Willa's buttocks; and Eugenia kept culturing the same microbe. Willa was delighted to have her lumps removed, and I was intrigued by the unusual microbes Eugenia cultured from Willa's tissue.

After much study, I was sure there were microbes in Willa's "panniculitis" tissue sections. I suspected the "granules" and the "balloon forms" had something to do with the acid-fast bacteria in Willa's ground-up tissue, and with the fungus cultured from her skin. But the pathologist insisted the tissue sections contained no microbes; and the granules and the large balloon bodies were not infectious agents. As far as the pathologist was concerned, Willa's case was closed.

While studying Willa's case, I investigated two other cases of "panniculitis." In both cases Eugenia found acid-fast bacteria in the ground-up tissue smears and she cultured microbes resembling "atypical" TB mycobacteria.

In 1965, I studied Juanita; a Latina with disfiguring panniculitis of the face, arms, trunk, and buttocks. At age 52, one side of her face was still beautiful but the other side was severely distorted with large, sunken areas of flesh. Eighteen years earlier, in 1947, she had a series of injections of female hormones and vitamins into her buttocks and arms. Shortly thereafter, she began to lose portions of skin fat and little red bumps appeared and slowly enlarged to form large areas of sunken skin. In 1960, red lesions appeared on her cheek. The lesions enlarged, the skin fat dissolved, and her beauty was destroyed.

A few acid-fast bacteria were found in Juanita's tissue

sections; and Eugenia cultured another strange microbe that could not be classified.

The new dermatology professor, Dr. J. Walter Wilson, suggested I inject Juanita's microbes into the foot pad of a mouse to determine the effect. After the injection the mouse remained healthy. Two months later the animal was killed to determine the effect. At autopsy, acid-fast bacteria were found in the foot pad that was injected; the rest of the mouse's body was free of acid-fast microbes.

Willa and Juanita's cases, along with two others, were published in the *Archives of Dermatology* in 1966[1]. It was an honor to have our work appear in this prestigious journal. Eugenia and I shared credits with Professor Wilson; and with Frank Swatek, Professor of Microbiology at Long Beach State.

Professor Wilson was also a world-famous dermatologist, as well as a medical expert in fungal skin diseases. He was highly supportive of my microbiologic research. However, he was concerned because I was finding so many "positive" specimens in panniculitis patients. He requested that I test skin specimens from other skin diseases in order to get some "negative" acid-fast bacteria specimens. This was necessary as an experimental "control" for my panniculitis research. He suggested I take some skin from one of the ward patients. Perhaps from Reuben. Reuben was dying of scleroderma, a disease "of unknown etiology" in which acid-fast microbes were never found.

Reuben's test was the true beginning of a scientific study that would consume me for the next three decades. My hunt for acid-fast bacteria would lift me into realms of scientific exhilaration, and into depths of despair and professional isolation.

With my scleroderma research and its consequences, I began to challenge the established dogma of modern medicine. I was an upstart dermatologist, new to the game of medical research and terribly intimidated by all the dermatologists who seemed to know so much more than I did. I had much to learn.

And much to unlearn.

References:

1. **Cantwell AR Jr, Craggs E, Swatek F, Wilson JW**: Unusual acid-fast bacteria in panniculitis. Arch Dermatol 94: 161-167, 1966.

CHAPTER FOUR

Reuben's Scleroderma

Reuben was a 37 year-old Mexican-American veteran and the youngest patient on the dermatology ward. I will never forget the look in his tormented eyes as he implored us to save him from the horrors of his relentless disease.

Scleroderma comes from Greek words meaning "hard skin." In scleroderma the body's fibrous tissue thickens and the skin toughens and constricts. It becomes difficult for patients to walk, use their hands, open their mouth, or even smile. The internal organs suffer as well. Reuben was becoming slowly encased in skin as hard as stone.

His suffering was made more severe by sores of the fingers and toes. Deep and painful ulcers pierced the flesh of his back and shoulders. Reuben was a pitiful sight, and with each passing month the skin ulcerations became larger and more numerous. There was little we could do to help him. None of us knew what caused scleroderma or how to cure it.

Scleroderma is closely related to two other diseases: rheumatoid arthritis and lupus erythematosus. All three diseases have similar immunologic abnormalities which link them together as so-called "connective tissue" diseases. It is believed that people with these three diseases are "allergic" and "autoimmune" to their own body tissue.

We all knew what would happen to Reuben. His internal organs would become more and more scarred, and when they could no longer function, Reuben's agony would end. Until that time, the nurses tried to make him as comfortable as possible.

Rueben agreed to let me take a piece of skin to test for germs. I chose a hard, stonelike area of skin next to a large ulcer on his back. The skin was deadened with an anesthestic and the area was carefully cleansed to minimize contamination from surface skin bacteria. The biopsy was over in moments. Half the tissue was sent to Eugenia Craggs in the TB lab; the other half to the pathologist.

By choosing Rueben's scleroderma skin tissue as a "control," I was set on a path of scientific study from which I could never veer, no matter how hard I tried. It was a path of destiny that led me into the secrets of scleroderma, cancer and AIDS, and finally into the origin of life itself.

When Eugenia received Reuben's tissue she added a little sterile saline water and mashed the specimen in a tissue grinder. Placing a tiny amount of the mashed tissue onto a glass slide, she then colored the tissue with the acid-fast stain. The stained material on the slide was covered with a thin glass coverslip, and a drop of microscope lens oil was placed on the coverslip. Eugenia put the slide onto her microscope and focused the oil-immersion lens that magnified Reuben's tissue preparation one thousand times.

After studying Reuben's tissue carefully, Eugenia phoned me at the dermatology clinic. "This is Eugenia in TB. The specimen on Reuben Gomez is positive for acid-fast bacteria."

"That's impossible," I said. "The skin is from a patient with scleroderma. There aren't any acid-fast bacteria in scleroderma!"

Eugenia was emphatic. "Well, I don't know anything about scleroderma, but I've been working in TB for years. And I know acid-fast rods when I see them. If you don't believe me, you can come over to the lab and look for yourself."

As I peered into Eugenia's microscope, I saw the red-stained acid-fast rods in Reuben's preliminary smear preparation. The red rods looked just like the mycobacteria that cause tuberculosis and leprosy. Eugenia had made a tremendous discovery. These microbes had to be important in Rueben's disease because it is never normal to find acid-fast bacteria in tissue.

What kind of mycobacteria were they? There was no way of telling until the microbes were grown in culture. All the acid-fast rods of the various species of mycobacteria can look the same. In order to determine the precise identification of Reuben's microbe we would have to wait until the culture was tested biochemically.

Eugenia had already planted Reuben's tissue on TB media but it could take weeks to grow. We had to be patient. In the meantime, I was confident the pathologist would see acid-fast bacteria in Reuben's tissue sections, just as Eugenia had seen them in Rueben's smear preparation. I was sure we had discovered the hidden cause of scleroderma.

My pipe dream was quickly burst by the pathologist who couldn't find acid-fast bacteria in Reuben's slides. I rechecked to be sure; there was none. Why were numerous acid-fast bacteria present in Eugenia's preparation, but not in the pathologist's tissue sections? Did the histologic process of chemically "fixing" the tissue somehow destroy Reuben's microbes or make them unstainable with the acid-fast dye?

There was another complication. A review of Rueben's

old medical records showed he was diagnosed with a
mild case of lung tuberculosis seven years before his
scleroderma began. As proof, there was a lab report
stating that *Mycobacterium tuberculosis* had been
cultured from his sputum. Were the acid-fast bacteria in
Reuben's scleroderma related to his old lung TB
infection? If so, I was confident Eugenia would be able
to grow *Mycobacterium tuberculosis* in her lab.

After several weeks of incubation, a microbe grew
from Reuben's tissue but it was not *Mycobacterium
tuberculosis*. Some of the bacteria were typical rod-
shaped acid-fast bacteria; but most of the forms were
round and "coccus-like" and not acid-fast. In addition,
some of Reuben's microbes were fungus-like and
produced long chains and filaments. Exactly what kind
of germ was growing? I had never seen such a peculiar
microbe with so many different forms! Eugenia suspected
Reuben's microbe might be an acid-fast fungus called
"Nocardia."

In the classification system of bacteria, the acid-fast
mycobacteria are closely related to fungi. "Myco" is the
Greek word for fungus. For the first half of this century,
microbiologists believed that only a few species of
mycobacteria were important in human and animal
disease. The two most common diseases caused by acid-
fast mycobacteria are tuberculosis (caused by *Mycobacterium tuberculosis*), and leprosy (caused by *Mycobacterium leprae*). In the textbooks it is always stated that
the germ of leprosy has never been cultured, but I later
learned that this "fact" is not true.

In the 1960s, mycobacteriologists began to recognize
other species of mycobacteria that cause disease in
human beings. These newly discovered species are
termed "atypical," "anonymous," or "unclassified"

mycobacteria. This was confusing to me because I was not well-trained in microbiology in medical school. However, in my scleroderma research, I soon discovered that most physicians are not well-versed in bacteriology. They simply do not have the necessary laboratory training and expertise to be knowledgeable in this field.

When the pathologist could not find acid-fast bacteria in Reuben's tissue, I wondered if Reuben's germ might be the leprosy germ. Leprosy mycobacteria are more difficult to stain than TB mycobacteria. And there are certain forms of leprosy in which acid-fast bacilli are extremely difficult to detect. Special acid-fast staining techniques have been devised to detect leprosy mycobacteria in tissue sections. I asked the technicians in the histology lab to try some of these special acid-fast stains on Reuben's sections.

One of the special leprosy stains proved successful. After many hours of microscopic examination, I found a few acid-fast rods in Reuben's skin. The red rods looked just like TB and leprosy bacilli.

Eugenia and other microbiologists could not precisely identify Reuben's microbe. They classified it as a possible "atypical" mycobacterium, or perhaps a fungus. I was learning that microbiology is not the exact science that I thought it was.

I was determined to prove that acid-fast bacteria were involved in scleroderma, and I had less than a year before my residency training would end at the VA. At the clinic there were two other veterans with scleroderma: a white man (age 42); and a black man (age 32). Compared to Reuben, their scleroderma was mild. I tested their skin, and I retested Reuben. Eugenia found acid-fast bacteria in all the specimens. The bacteria were all impossible to classify precisely. None were "typical"

TB mycobacteria.

When my residency ended in the fall of 1965, I joined the staff of a large clinic in Hollywood, where I have practiced ever since. I continued to attend the weekly dermatology conferences at the Long Beach VA, and always visited Eugenia's lab to check on the scleroderma cultures. Her boss began to resent the time and effort Eugenia devoted to the scleroderma work. He complained the research was unauthorized, and he was annoyed when she shipped our cultures to other microbiologists at other institutions for expert identification. He bristled when Eugenia's name appeared (along with Frank Swatek, Professor of Microbiology at Long Beach State College) on our paper on panniculitis, published by the *Archives of Dermatology* in 1966[1]. I was beginning to understand the peculiarities of hospital and medical politics, and the fragility of biomedical egos.

At this time I had already developed a reputation as a kooky dermatologist who was finding mysterious acid-fast bacteria in diseases "of unknown etiology." Kiddingly, the derm residents at the VA used to greet me with, "Hey, Alan! Found any more little red bugs lately?"

Professor Wilson was a great source of encouragement. He was a powerful force in dermatology, having served as President of the American Academy of Dermatology and having authored many scientific papers, as well as a popular textbook on fungal diseases.

On February 9, 1966, Dr. Wilson arranged to have Reuben presented to The Los Angeles Metropolitan Dermatologic Society. We showed color photographs of the acid-fast bacteria that were found in his scleroderma tissue. Reuben's case was recorded in the *Archives of Dermatology* in November 1966[2]. When asked what kind of organism we cultured, I responded: "I must emphasize that the growth of this organism was scant. Many of the forms were non-acid-fast, and at times the bacillus tended to branch like a Nocardia (a fungus); we are at a loss as to how it should be classified."

Mercifully, Reuben died a year later. Lenora, my favorite nurse at the VA, called me at my Hollywood office to tell me of his passing. She was a funny lady who always lightened up the clinic staff with her off-color jokes. Lenora was savvy enough to know I was gay, and practically had to hit me over the head to make me realize she was a lesbian. How would I know? I had never known a lesbian, and I never would have suspected Lenora if she hadn't told me.

"Hi Doll," she said. "I'm sorry to tell you that Reuben died last night. I know you wanted to be notified in case they were going to do an autopsy. But there isn't going to be one. The family is in Arizona. They refused to sign for the autopsy and the body is being shipped there for burial."

"Oh, shoot," I moaned. "I can't believe they didn't get an autopsy. We have to get more skin biopsies for testing! His case is so important." Strangely, I felt no sadness for Reuben's passing. His death was a blessing.

Lenora detected my disappointment. She knew how hard I had studied the microbes that were slowly killing Reuben. "His body was shipped up to East LA for embalming. Why don't you call the mortician? I'm sure he'll let you take some skin."

I thought she was joking, but she wasn't. She persisted. "Do you want some of his skin, or don't you? Why don't you at least try?" I jotted down the number and address, and thanked her for her bizarre idea. I never would have thought of it myself.

The afternoon was overcast and drizzly as I drove from Hollywood to the mortuary in East LA. I wondered what madness was overtaking me in my desire to uncover the secrets of scleroderma. Nobody in his right mind did research like this.

The mortician acted like my request for skin was an everyday occurrence. As long as I didn't take the biopsies from any place that showed, he didn't care. The family in Arizona wasn't planning on opening Reuben's casket, but just in case they changed their mind, he didn't want any trouble. I quickly took half a dozen large and deep skin samples. I would never have done such a thing to Reuben while he was alive; it would have been a cruel and savage act. But now that he was dead, Reuben still had something to offer the world; I would make sure of that. I thanked the mortician, offered a quick prayer for Reuben, and hurried out into the rain.

The next day I sent a skin specimen to Carville, Louisiana, to the U.S. Public Health Hospital, which specializes in the treatment of leprosy (Hansen's disease). Another specimen was sent to Ruth Gordon at Rutgers.

Several months later I received a report from Richard E. Mansfield MD, Chief of the Laboratory Branch at Carville. He wrote: "The reason it took so long to get the final report was that a rapid-growing, acid-fast bacterium was cultured from the tissue you sent. We have found this to be *Mycobacterium fortuitum*. We have just received confirmation from the National Centers for Communicable Disease in Atlanta, Georgia. Acid-fast bacteria were found on rare slides. Further recuts are being made and I will send you a marked slide where definite acid-fast rods can be identified." Doctor Mansfield expressed some concern as to whether the tissue might be contaminated, or whether the acid-fast bacteria might have developed after the scleroderma process took hold. I decided not to tell him how I got the samples. Ruth Gordon wrote that she also had cultured *Mycobacterium fortuitum* and remarked, "We had better luck in recognizing it than some cultures you have sent us."

Mycobacterium fortuitum is an "atypical" species of mycobacteria that can cause TB in humans. There was no way it could have been a contaminant. I was confident it was the same acid-fast microbe that Eugenia had detected a year and a half earlier. Why was it so difficult to recognize it at that time? Eugenia frequently cultured *M. fortuitum* in her TB lab. Perhaps Reuben's acid-fast microbe had changed as he neared death, so that the identity and classification of the microbe were now more obvious.

From my work at the VA with Eugenia I learned one important thing: microbes change form. Sometimes they appear one way, sometimes another. And they could fool the experts. The appearance of the microbe depended on what it was fed in the laboratory. In the textbooks of microbiology the classification of organisms was simple and straightforward. But in reality, it was not that way at all.

I enjoyed talking about my scleroderma research to friends who seemed interested in my tales of medical adventure at the VA. A gay friend told me about a psychic who believed TB germs were involved in scleroderma; and a dermatologist at the VA heard about a physician who claimed scleroderma was an infection caused by acid-fast bacteria.

I thought I was alone in my scleroderma research. Now I discovered there were two others. I had to find out more about them. Perhaps they could tell me about those strange little red bugs that turned Reuben's skin to stone and finally killed him.

References:

1. **Cantwell AR Jr, Craggs E, Swatek F, Wilson JW**: Unusual acid- fast bacteria in panniculitis. Arch Dermatol 94: 161-167, 1966.

2. **Cantwell AR Jr, Wilson JW**: Scleroderma with ulceration secondary to atypical mycobacteria. Arch Dermatol 94: 663- 664, 1966.

CHAPTER FIVE

Livingston's *Progenitor Cryptocides*

During the mid-1960s when I immersed myself in my scleroderma studies, I also began to investigate the world of the occult. I yearned to discover the meaning and purpose of life. It was difficult to fully accept my sexual identity because of the strong cultural, social, and religious taboos against homosexuality; and I could no longer find spiritual solace within the anti-gay Roman Catholic church.

During this period of emotional chaos Eugenia Craggs mentioned that she knew a woman astrologer who was interested in our scleroderma research. She told Eugenia she would be happy to do my horoscope for free. I knew nothing about astrology and I was curious about the subject. In the 1960s "the age of Aquarius" and "what's your sign?" were the rage. As requested, I sent my birthdate and the time and place of birth to Judy Cooper. A week later I received my horoscope chart along with a "reading."

I was fascinated with Judy's reading and with her unorthodox ideas and beliefs. I wanted to know how she was able to interpret my personal life through astrology. Judy wrote that she would help me learn astrology, but warned that if I began to seriously study the subject, I would not be able to dismiss it. Throwing caution to the wind, I avidly began my investigation of the planetary art of the ancients.

The more I understood how astrology "worked," the more intrigued I became. I learned how to construct horoscope charts and practiced giving readings to family and friends. The study of my own chart convinced me I was not on the planet "by accident." My worldly desires, my emotional needs, my spiritual quest, all seemed related to the symbolic messages represented by the positions of the planets and the signs in my horoscope. I was amazed how the planetary configuration at the moment of my birth seemed to correlate with the kind of life experiences I was seeking on this planet. There is no need to prove astrology to anyone. It is part of the Hindu and Buddhist religion and believed by millions of people. Personally, I know there is spiritual and worldly truth in astrology because I have studied it.

Astrology has helped me accept my nature as a somewhat eccentric human being. Through astrology I have discovered my purpose in life and I am content knowing I am part of the divine plan. And I no longer brood over the fact that I am not "normal" (whatever that is).

Around the same time I began to study astrology, I also became interested in the writings of Edgar Cayce.

I first heard about Edgar Cayce through my friend Harlan. He was reading about scleroderma in a book called *THERE IS A RIVER*,[1] and phoned me. "Guess what?" he asked excitedly. "I'm reading a book about Edgar Cayce and he says there are TB germs in scleroderma. That's exactly what you've been telling me about your own research."

"Who's Edgar Cayce?" I asked.

"He's a psychic who goes into a trance and taps into the universal consciousness. He tells people about their illness and how to treat it. Actually, he's been dead since 1945. This is the second book I've read about him. The other is *THE SLEEPING PROPHET*[2]. You should read it."

"Harlan. I'm not sure I know what you're talking about. Just tell me what he says about scleroderma and TB germs."

Harlan read from Tom Sugrue's book about a woman with severe scleroderma who sought medical advice from Casey in 1937. In his psychic state Cayce saw "disturbances caused by the effect of the tubercle (TB) activity to the superficial circulation." The disturbances involved the lymph circulation and the glandular system. As a result, the woman's white blood cells were unable to suppress the TB microbes that were active in scleroderma.

When I read more books about the "sleeping prophet" and his strange beliefs, I discovered there are 14, 000 recorded psychic readings. Over 9000 are on the subject of health and disease. The other readings cover such esoteric subjects as psychic phenomena, dreams, astrology, reincarnation, karmic relationships, Atlantis, and future world predictions.

I contacted The Association for Research and Enlightenment (A.R.E.) which makes the Cayce material available to the general public. The A.R.E. referred me to two physicians, Bill McGarey and his wife Gladys, who were investigating Cayce's healing methods at their clinic in Phoenix, Arizona. The McGareys were astonished that I had confirmed Casey's psychic pronouncement of tuberculosis bacteria in scleroderma.

The A.R.E. also sent me the medical files on scleroderma, along with Bill McGarey's "Commentary." According to Cayce, scleroderma is caused by a malfunction of the glands of the body. This produces a deficiency which "creates a lack of nutrition in the circulation of the skin itself." Eventually the flow of the lymph circulation becomes disturbed. The lymphatic channels become inflamed and actually create TB germs. These TB microbes further damage the circulation of the skin and produce scleroderma.

I immediately took issue with Cayce. His idea that scleroderma TB germs are created in the disturbed tissue cells was medical heresy. Microbiology teaches that microbes originate from outside the body, never from within. Even Bill McGarey thought Cayce's view of TB scleroderma microbes was peculiar. In *EDGAR CAYCE ON HEALING*, Bill comments: "The tubercle bacillus is in this instance a product of the body itself, not a secondary invader. A few medical theorists have implied that viruses derive sometimes from still vital chromosomal material left over from cellular breakdowns. But nowhere has the idea been proposed that the body (itself) may produce an acid-fast bacillus, or any type of bacteria, for that matter."[3]

Putting this controversy aside, I was interested in Cayce's ideas on health and healing. A quote from Casey in the *EDGAR CAYCE HANDBOOK FOR HEALTH* provides a concise summary of his philosophy:

". . . all strength, all healing of every nature is the changing of the vibrations from within — the attuning of the divine within the living tissue of a body to Creative Energies. This alone is healing. Whether it is accomplished by the use of drugs, the knife, or what-not, it is the attuning of the atomic structure of the living cellular force to its spiritual heritage."[4]

Cayce's philosophy was provocative, but he was

obviously wrong about the origin of TB bacteria in scleroderma. It proved he did not understand the elementary "facts" of microbiology. Or so I thought.

For many years Cayce's scleroderma error bugged me. Two decades later I began to realize that Cayce may have been on to something vitally important in the understanding of disease pathology. In tapping into the "universal mind or consciousness" for his medical diagnoses, Cayce may have zeroed into alternative microbiologic concepts espoused by scientists like Antoine Bechamp, Wilhelm Reich, and others. It may well be that Cayce was correct in his psychic pronouncement that microbes can originate in diseased cells and altered tissue. . . but this is getting ahead of the story.

Edgar Cayce (1877-1945) was a simple, uneducated man with an unprecedented gift for clairvoyance and an uncanny knowledge of the causes of sickness and disease. His psychic readings of the 1930s were prophetic of the current "holistic medicine" movement, which stresses that man is a being composed of "body, mind and spirit."

Privately, I was entranced with Cayce, but his ideas on scleroderma were of little use to me. In my scientific writings I could never publicize Cayce's belief that TB microbes were involved in scleroderma.

For a short while, I was alone on my research path. But I had the secret company of an inexplicable, long-dead psychic. Soon I would meet a woman doctor who would understand my scleroderma discoveries. Her critics labelled her a medical Dragon Lady, a quack and a charlaton. But she became my friend, my teacher, and my scientific guru. And she profoundly affected my life.

After I met her I was no longer alone.

———

In the spring of 1968 Roy Averill, one of the dermatology

residents at the VA, cornered me after the derm conference and said, "You won't believe this, but I was in San Diego this past weekend and I heard a physician being interviewed on the radio. She spoke about finding acid-fast bacteria in scleroderma and cancer. She practices in San Diego. You should have no trouble finding her phone number in the book. Her name is Livingston. Virginia Livingston."

I telephoned. Virginia was delighted to hear about my scleroderma research, and I was thrilled to hear about hers. She invited me to San Diego to meet her and Afton, her physician husband.

Virginia deluged me with a pile of published papers that she had written with a variety of dermatologists, pathologists, microbiologists, and microscopists. I instantly learned about dozens of other researchers whose work was intimately connected to Virginia's research, and to mine.

Virginia was born in 1906. Her father, H. H. Wuerthele MD, practiced in a small coal mining town in Pennsylvania. As a young girl she carried his medical bag on house calls; and by age 10 she was assisting in home deliveries. Virginia was determined to be a physician, even though it was an unusual profession for a woman in those days.

After graduation from New York University Medical School she became the first woman doctor to be accepted as an internal medicine resident at a New York City hospital. Virginia claims she successfully pressured City officials until they reluctantly granted her a position — at a prison hospital in Brooklyn.

The position was hardly prestigious, but Virginia was enthralled with the unusual infectious disease cases she encountered at the hospital. Her training, especially with tuberculosis and leprosy cases, proved invaluable. A few years later her leprosy experience allowed Virginia to make the most important discovery of her career. While examining a school nurse with scleroderma and painful ulcerations of the fingers and nose, Virginia was reminded of the leprosy patients she had treated at the prison hospital. Instinctively she took a pin and tested the nurse's skin reaction to pain. Curiously, some scleroderma areas had no feeling.

Virginia tested the scleroderma skin to determine if acid-fast bacilli were present, just like she had been taught to do in leprosy cases. She scraped tiny bits of the nurse's skin onto a glass slide and stained the preparation with an acid-fast dye. Virginia knew that if acid-fast leprosy or TB microbes were present in the nurse's tissue the stain would color them red. After placing a drop of oil on the stained material, she carefully examined the tissue for acid-fast bacteria. *In the flakes of the scleroderma skin tissue Virginia found the red-stained, rod-shaped, acid-fast microbes that looked exactly like leprosy and TB mycobacteria!*

Virginia's discovery was brilliant. But the discovery was the easy part. The hard part would be to get the medical world to accept it.

In studying scleroderma, Virginia allied herself to two women: Camille Mermod, a pathologist; and Eva Brodkin, a dermatologist. The three physicians proved that microbes existed in the tissue of scleroderma, and they were successful in culturing bacteria from the scleroderma skin samples. Virginia injected the scleroderma bacteria into chicks and guinea pigs. The chicks died, and the skin of the guinea pigs hardened like scleroderma. Some guinea pigs developed cancer. This was very unusual, because guinea pigs are highly resistant to cancer.

In July 1947, *The Journal of the Medical Society of New Jersey* published Virginia's paper, "Etiology of scleroderma; A preliminary report," co-authored by Eva Brodkin and Camille Mermod[5]. Five cases of scleroderma with acid-fast bacteria were reported. The scleroderma organism was tentatively named "sclerobacillus Wuerthele-Caspe," pending further bacteriologic studies.

Besides being employed as a school physician, Virginia led a busy life as the wife of a noted chemist, Joseph Caspe, and as the mother of an adopted baby daughter. Nevertheless, she managed to find time to pursue her microbiologic research. The ability of the scleroderma microbe to produce cancer in animals led Virginia to suspect that a similar microbe might also be involved in human cancer. She avidly searched for acid-fast bacteria in cancer tissue that she colored with the acid-fast stain. She cultured various cancer tumors and carefully examined the bacteria that grew from the tumors. And she tested the cancer bacteria to determine if they were acid-fast. By the time the New Jersey *Journal* published her scleroderma paper, Virginia had already discovered acid-fast microbes in cancer.

Virginia surrounded herself with talented scientists who aided tremendously in her cancer research. Although over 70 years of age, Roy Allen was still an expert microscopist and histologist. He possessed a remarkable collection of microscopes, one of which could magnify tissue 2500 times. (Ordinary microscopes magnify only about 1000 times.) In addition, he possessed excellent camera equipment designed for microphotography.

In "The microscopy of micro-organisms associated with neoplasms (cancer),"[6] published in the August 1948 issue of *The New York Microscopical Bulletin*, Roy

Allen presents illustrations of the cancer microbe and explains how it can be identified in tissue stained with the special acid-fast stain. He stresses that the cancer microbe is "pleomorphic," indicating it has more than one appearance. The microbe can be rod-shaped or coccus (round) shaped. The germ can be stained acid-fast (red) or non-acid-fast (blue). The non-acid-fast round coccal forms appear as single, double, or as densely packed round forms. These coccus forms vary in size from 1 micron down to the smallest size the eye can see (0.2 microns). The microbes live inside the cancer cells (intracellular) and outside the cells (extracellular). Roy Allen claimed that every patholologist had seen the cancer microbe, but had failed to interpret its true nature.

The tiniest, barely visible forms of the cancer microbe are "filterable" and virus-sized. Viruses are smaller than bacteria. Microbiologists use special laboratory filters to separate viruses and bacteria. Bacterial filters have pore openings which allow the smaller viruses to pass through, but not the larger bacteria. Laboratory filters are designed like a kitchen sieve which allows small dirt and sand particles to pass through, but not larger substances, such as grains of rice or peas.

Virginia believes the tiny filterable forms of the cancer microbe are related to cancer viruses. These virus forms of the cancer microbe are too small to be seen with a regular microscope. However, they can be visualized with the powerful electron microscope which magnifies 60,000 times, or higher. James Hillier of Princeton used the electron microscope to photograph the virus forms of Virginia's cancer microbe at a magnification of 30,000 times. Virginia obtained these pure virus forms by filtering bacterial cultures obtained from cancer tumors.

In order to prove that bacteria originate from these filtered (bacteria-free) cultures, Virginia prepared multiple vials of bacteria-free filtrates from a single cancer microbe culture. Every few days, one of the bottles was opened and the filtrate examined. With the proper growth media and the passage of time, Virginia could induce the cancer bacteria to reappear in the filtered (bacteria-free) fluid. This was proof that cancer bacteria originated from submicroscopic viruses.

During the five years (1948-1953) that Virginia worked in her Newark cancer laboratory she collaborated with John A. Anderson, Professor of Bacteriology at Rutgers University; Lawrence W. Smith, a well-known pathologist affiliated with Newark Presbyterian Hospital; and Eleanor Alexander-Jackson, a microbiologist from Cornell University Medical School.

By 1950 the group had enough experimental and research data to present their work to other scientists. In December 1950, *The American Journal of Medical Sciences* was the first major medical journal to publish Virginia's cancer research. The paper entitled, "Cultural properties and pathogenicity of certain microorganisms obtained from various proliferative and neoplastic diseases,"[7] was co-authored by Virginia, John Anderson, James Hillier, Roy Allen, Lawrence Smith, and Eleanor Alexander-Jackson. The eleven-page article contains an electron microscopic picture of the virus form of the cancer microbe magnified 31,000 times; microphotographs of the cancer bacteria cultured from the blood and bone marrow of cancer patients; and pictures of diseased lungs and kidneys of animals experimentally infected with the cancer microbe. A classic description of the cancer microbe was provided:

"These organisms, which appear primarily as small

acid-fast granules in young cultures and which tend to become non-acid-fast in the larger forms present in old cultures, may exhibit a number of types, such as: a) minute filterable granules beyond the limits of visibility of the light microscope; b) larger granules approximately the size of ordinary cocci, readily seen with the light microscope; c) still larger round globoidal forms; d) rod-like forms with irregular staining; and e) occasionally globoidal forms which appear to undergo polar budding."

When I first met Virginia she wanted me to get involved in the cancer work and she even offered me a job at her clinic. But I enjoyed being a dermatologist and I didn't want to work exclusively with cancer patients. I treasured Virginia's friendship and her outstanding research accomplishments. However, it was distressing for me to learn that the medical community had labelled Virginia a quack.

Virginia's discovery of a microbe in cancer should have been heralded as the major medical discovery of the twentieth century. Instead, it destroyed her credibility in the medical community.

Virginia's controversial cancer research stirred up trouble with powerful people in the American cancer establishment. The details of her confrontation with the establishment are provided in her autobiographical books *CANCER: A NEW BREAKTHROUGH* (1972), and *THE CONQUEST OF CANCER* (1984)[8, 9].

Virginia could never keep silent about the cancer microbe. The work was too important. She constantly fought the cancer experts, who insisted that bacteria were not important in cancer. Every time she spoke about the cancer microbe, she was inevitably pegged as just another crazy California quack.

I didn't want to get involved in Virginia's conquest of cancer. Even if I wanted to help her, I couldn't. I worked for an "establishment" institution. Experimental cancer treatments were forbidden unless they were approved by a special committee. I already had a reputation for harboring strange ideas about scleroderma, and I didn't want to get caught up in the cancer microbe controversy and antagonize the medical establishment the way Virginia did.

Through Virginia I was introduced to Dan Kelso, a Los Angeles microbiologist. Dan was enthusiastic about Virginia's ideas and agreed to help with my scleroderma cultures. Finding Dan was miraculous. He was often able to culture the scleroderma microbe from skin tissue samples, and over the past twenty years we have collaborated on many scientific papers on scleroderma, cancer, and AIDS.

In spite of Virginia's encouragement and Dan's expertise, my scleroderma research was hitting some snags. I spent countless hours searching for acid-fast bacilli in the tissue sections of new scleroderma cases but frequently I was unable to find them. I knew I could never convince other dermatologists that acid-fast mycobacteria caused scleroderma unless the microbes were quickly and easily found in the scleroderma tissue sections. Busy doctors simply do not have the time to spend hours searching for scleroderma bacteria with "negative" results.

I expected Dan to culture acid-fast bacteria like Eugenia had done. But instead he cultured non-acid-fast cocci resembling ordinary *Staphylococcus epidermidis*, a common microbe that lives on the skin and a common laboratory "contaminant." No physician or microbiologist would ever believe that this microbe was the cause of scleroderma!

In other instances Dan cultured microbes composed of cocci and rods. He identified these "coccobacilli" as Corynebacteria (also known as "diphtheroids"), another common skin microbe and laboratory contaminant. To make matters worse, most of the cultured microbes were not acid-fast. Frequently we saw tiny acid-fast "granules." But I needed to find acid-fast rods, not granules. Pathologists were always impressed with acid-fast rods, but never with acid-fast "granules" of dubious origin.

It was vital to show medical journal editors pictures of acid-fast rods in scleroderma tissue. They wanted to see not just one or two acid-fast rods, but many. A few rods could indicate that the tissue was contaminated with acid-fast bacteria. Tap water, even distilled water, was known to contain a few contaminating acid-fast myco-bacteria that could work their way onto the slides. Without showing definite acid-fast bacteria in the tissue of every scleroderma case, it would be exceedingly difficult to prove that acid-fast bacteria caused scleroderma.

I kept hounding Dan for the precise identity of the germs he cultured. Often the microbes changed form, indicating they were "pleomorphic." It was difficult for Dan to be sure. In order to classify microbes they had to be "stable," not "pleomorphic." We soon discovered that scleroderma microbes grew best in liquid, rather than solid laboratory media.

I insisted Dan keep the liquid cultures for weeks; and this posed a new set of problems because the longer a lab culture is kept, the more likely it is to get contami-nated. In most labs, "routine" cultures are discarded after a few days. But scleroderma microbes grow slowly. As the scleroderma cultures age, the microbes tend to become more bizarre and more pleomorphic. Microbiologists are often reluctant to identify "old" cultures that are pleomorphic.

I wanted Dan to grow easily identifiable acid-fast bacteria which could be "classified" as definite mycobacteria. Virginia stressed that the scleroderma and cancer microbes were "intermittently acid-fast." And without that red-colored hallmark it was impossible for Dan and me to be sure we had cultured the correct scleroderma microbe.

From Dan and Eugenia I learned valuable lessons that are not discussed in microbiology textbooks. I learned that microbes can vary considerably in their appearance. Their appearance or "morphology" changes as the culture ages. The form of a microbe can also change, depending on the laboratory "media" used to culture the microbe.

I discovered that certain "pure" cultures of staphylococci (which were supposed to contain only round forms) could also contain "rod" forms. According to the textbooks this is impossible. But in actual practice it is true. I learned that bacteria identified as "cocci" could transform into rod-shaped "coccobacilli" when transferred from one growth media to another; and coccobacilli could be tranformed into "pure" cocci by changing the laboratory media.

Many microbiologists do not accept what is plain to see in their laboratories. And most biologists do not accept the concept and the reality of bacterial pleomorphism. Bacterial pleomorphism goes against the inviolate (and unnatural) "classification" system invented by microbiologists. Microbiologists ignore the fact that microbes frequently do not behave "according to the book." In reality, microbes react as they want to react.

In reality, they are often "unclassifiable."

It took me a decade to unlearn the "facts" I was taught in medical school. My inability to comprehend the true nature of microbes prevented me from understanding the infectious process in scleroderma. Physicians and microbiologists believe that a coccus is always a coccus; a rod is always a rod. A rod never becomes a coccus, or vice-versa. My research proved these concepts were totally incorrect!

Virginia was labelled a crazy scientist because she saw cancer bacteria that cancer experts would not see. She knew that cancer bacteria resembled "regular" staphylococci or "diphtheroid" coccobacilli, or yeast, or fungi. And the cancer microbe had an invisible "virus" phase that could not be detected microscopically.

Virginia's cancer microbe violated the established laws of microbiology. The microbiologists were peeved when Virginia audaciously named the scleroderma microbe ("*sclerobacillus Wuerthele-Caspe*") after herself. They were angered because only established committies of microbiological experts have the authority to name microbes. Then when Virginia discovered the so-called cancer microbe she named it "*Progenitor cryptocides*" — the ancestral hidden killer of cancer. The experts fumed! How dare this quack doctor name a cancer microbe that does not exist?

Where did Virginia learn about pleomorphism? Certainly not in medical school. How could she write with such confidence and authority about the cancer microbe when the entire concept was scientific heresy?

In her earliest 1950 cancer paper[7] Virginia searched the biomedical literature to prove that microbes did tricks that were unheard of in microbiology. However, as brilliant as Virginia was, there were limits to her ability to explain esoteric microbiologic memorabilia that she had never learned in medical school.

After having met Virginia I soon met her best friend, Eleanor, who was visiting from New York. Eleanor was the power behind the throne. She was the microbiologist who introduced Virginia to little-known secrets of microbiology that were known to only a few physicians.

I liked Eleanor Alexander-Jackson the moment I met her. Unlike Virginia, Eleanor was reserved and shy. She had a wealth of information to impart about the cancer microbe, but I didn't understand most of it. She also presented me with her scientific papers on TB and leprosy.

As my frustration with the scleroderma work mounted, I became more interested in Eleanor's research on bacterial pleomorphism. There was no way I could understand the scleroderma and the cancer microbe without learning about pleomorphism. Virginia understood the concept quickly. I was slow; it took years to sink in.

When I finally understood it, I knew I had to follow Virginia and Eleanor in their quest to conquer cancer.

I had to study the cancer microbe.

References:

1. **Sugrue T**: *There is a River.* Holt, Rinehart and Winston, New York, 1942.

2. **Stearn J**: *Edgar Cayce: The Sleeping Prophet.* Doubleday & Co., Garden City, New York, 1967.

3. **Carter ME and McGarey WA**: *Edgar Cayce on*

Healing. Paperback Library, Coronet Communications, Inc., New York, 1972.

4. **Reilly HJ and Brod RH**: *The Edgar Cayce Handbook for Health Through Drugless Therapy.* Macmillan Publishing Co., New York, 1975.

5. **Wuerthele-Caspe V, Brodkin E, Mermod, C**: Etiology of scleroderma. Preliminary clinical report. J Med Soc New Jersey 44: 256-259, 1947.

6. **Allen RM**: The microscopy of micro-organisms associated with neoplasms. New York Microscopical Soc Bull 2: 19-26, 1948.

7. **Wuerthele-Caspe V, Alexander-Jackson E, Anderson JA, et al**: Cultural properties and pathogenicity of certain microorganisms obtained from various proliferative and neoplastic diseases. Am J Med Sci 220: 638-648, 1950.

8. **Livingston VWC**: *Cancer: A New Breakthrough.* Nash Publishing Corp., Los Angeles, 1972.

9. **Livingston-Wheeler V, Addeo EG**: *The Conquest of Cancer.* Franklin Watts, New York, 1984.

CHAPTER SIX

Alexander-Jackson and Pleomorphism

Eleanor Alexander-Jackson began studying the microbe of tuberculosis in 1928. She quickly discovered unusual growth forms of the tubercle bacillus that were never recorded in the textbooks. In 1934, the year I was born, she received her doctorate degree in Bacteriology. The prestigious *American Review of Tuberculosis* subsequently published a portion of her doctorate thesis on strange-looking "S" forms of the TB microbe.

Eleanor was a master in detecting and growing TB mycobacteria. She devised a new staining method (the Alexander-Jackson triple stain)[1] for detecting non-acid-fast forms of mycobacteria in tissue specimens; and also concocted a laboratory medium (Alexander-Jackson sensitive peptone broth) that made mycobacteria grow better and faster. In 1941 she joined the staff of Cornell Medical College as an expert TB microbiologist.

Although the red-stained, acid-fast rod form of the tubercle bacillus is the classic hallmark for the identification of the TB microbe, Eleanor was particularly interested in the blue-stained, non-acid-fast microbes she frequently observed in TB cultures and in the infected tissues of TB patients. In addition, she was intrigued by the tiny "granules;" the larger "coccus-like" forms; and the still larger "globoid" forms of the tubercle bacillus. They were all part of the many faces of the tuberculosis germ. Eleanor could never understand why microbiologists paid no attention to these mutant, pleomorphic forms that were so important in tuberculosis infection.

Eleanor was encouraged by a few other researchers who were equally passionate about pleomorphism. Soon after Robert Koch discovered the tubercle bacillus in 1882, other microbiologists began to notice "granules" contained within the rod-shaped tubercle bacillus. The granules were also frequently found scattered about in TB cultures and in infected TB tissue. Beginning in 1908 Hans Much wrote extensively about TB granules and they eventually became known as "Much's granules."[2] The precise nature of the granules remains controversial to this day.

Scientists who experimented with TB granules believed the granules were part of a "life cycle" of the constantly changing TB germ. In 1910 Fontes proved the granules were filterable[3]. The tiniest filter-passing forms were too small to be seen microscopically and became known as the TB "virus." When injected into guinea pigs the granules caused immune system disease and tuberculosis.

The scientists observed some granules enlarge to the size of ordinary-looking cocci — and watched other granules sprout into typical acid-fast rods. Eleanor was the first to write about a slimy "zooglear" matrix in which the TB granules are formed[4]. Mycobacteriologists also knew that highly virulent and deadly TB microbes could degenerate into harmless non-acid-fast cocci and into "diphtheroid" coccobacilli which looked exactly like common staphylococci and corynebacteria.

All this granule business bored most physicians, who couldn't understand why people like Eleanor were wasting time on such matters. But a few dedicated researchers knew the TB granules were important, and might even be involved in cancer. In 1928 H. C. Sweany proposed that filterable and granular forms of tubercle bacilli could cause Hodgkin's disease, a form of cancer[5-7].

In 1931, Pla y Armengol, a Barcelona scientist, claimed that the TB granules were the forms which attacked the cells and initiated the TB infection. He also grew pleomorphic TB microbes which looked exactly like fungi[8].

In a series of papers published in the 1930s, Ralph Mellon, Lawrence Beinhauer, and L. W. Fisher declared that mutant TB microbes caused Hodgkin's disease and sarcoidosis (a lung disease resembling tuberculosis). They also proposed a "life cycle" for TB microbes. In the "cycle" were acid-fast and non-acid-fast microbes that looked exactly like common staphylococci, corynebacteria, and fungi[9-11].

Despite all this research showing the pleomorphism of the tubercle bacillus, medical students are still taught that the microbe exists solely as an acid-fast, rod-shaped bacterium. As a result of this rigid and incorrect thinking, physicians are taught to recognize only the "acid-fast rod form" of the TB microbe. The tragic result of this erroneous teaching is that pathologists are not trained to recognize pleomorphic bacteria that produce serious human disease, such as cancer, AIDS, and other immunologic diseases.

Eleanor knew all the disguises of the TB germ. She knew that mutant forms of tubercle bacilli caused troublesome TB infection. She noted that when acid-fast rods disappeared from the sputum of recovering TB patients, the rods transformed into non-acid-fast pleomorphic forms. Conversely, when the pleomorphic forms reconverted to acid-fast rods the patient's TB became "active" again. TB germs did not die easily; they survived by transforming into pleomorphic forms.

In certain TB cases it is impossible to find acid-fast bacilli in the infected tissue. Yet even in these "negative" cases, it is sometimes possible to culture the TB microbe from the infected tissue. Furthermore, guinea pigs inoculated with "negative" TB tissue can occasionally become infected with TB. All this is possible because unrecognized pleomorphic TB microbes are present in the "negative" tissue. Under appropriate conditions these pleomorphic microbes transform into typical acid-fast bacilli.

For over ten years Eleanor struggled to prove that the seed of TB infection was hidden in the granules and in the coccoid forms, and even in the slime of the "zooglear plasmodium." In 1945 this TB research was published in Eleanor's paper entitled "A hitherto undemonstrated zoogleal form of *Mycobacterium tuberculosis*."[4]

Eleanor made valuable contributions to the microbiology of tuberculosis, but few people cared about her research. Later, when she began to lecture and write about the cancer microbe, powerful people in medical science paid close attention to Eleanor. Some of these people conspired to destroy her career as a research scientist.

———

After discovering acid-fast bacteria in scleroderma, Virginia Livingston injected the microbes into chickens and guinea pigs to determine the effect. The chickens became sickly and died; and some guinea pigs developed cancer tumors. Virginia stained the cancerous tissue with the acid-fast stain, and discovered the cancer microbe.

A colleague told Virginia about Eleanor's TB and leprosy research at Cornell. The two women met in 1947

and formed a scientific association and a friendship
which has lasted over 40 years. When Eleanor carefully
scrutinized the scleroderma and cancer slides and
cultures, she was amazed by the similarity of Virginia's
microbes to the TB and leprosy mycobacteria she had
studied. In scleroderma and cancer, Eleanor saw the
pleomorphic granules, coccoid forms, and globoids that
pathologists and microbiologists always ignored.

Eleanor agreed to help with Virginia's research. She
taught Virginia how to color cancer microbes with her
special "A-J" acid-fast staining technique. When Eleanor
filtered the cancer bacteria cultures, she showed Virginia
the tiny acid-fast granules in the filtrate. The cancer
microbe was filterable, just like the tubercle bacillus.
Eleanor contacted James Hillier, who photographed the
filterable, submicroscopic forms with his powerful
electron microscope at Princeton. Hillier's superb
electron microscopic photographs of Eleanor's slimy
zoogleal forms and TB granules had helped her win the
A. Cressy Morrison Prize in Natural Science in 1944 for
her TB research.

As the cancer work started in earnest, so did the
problems. No one bothered Eleanor while she confined
her research to TB and leprosy. However, when Eleanor's
superiors at Cornell Medical College heard she was
collaborating in cancer microbe research with a controversial woman doctor from New Jersey, that was another
matter. The college brass told Virginia to stay away from
the lab at Cornell, and Eleanor feared she might lose her
job.

During this time Eleanor was finishing a research
project in which she succeeded in culturing pleomorphic
acid-fast bacteria from the blood of leprosy patients.
When she injected the leprosy germs into white mice, the

animals developed skin ulcers.

Eleanor's leprosy research was highly unorthodox because microbiologists believe it is impossible to grow leprosy germs in laboratory culture. Eleanor's leprosy microbes showed pleomorphic forms (granules, coccoid and globoids forms, and diphtheroid-like organisms) similar to pleomorphic TB mycobacteria. James Hillier photographed the virus forms of the leprosy microbe at a magnification of 15,000. Eleanor's research was published in *The International Journal of Leprosy* in 1951 ("The cultivation and morphological study of a pleomorphic organism from the blood of leprosy patients") [12].

Eleanor had performed the impossible task of culturing the microbe of leprosy. She emphasized that pleomorphic leprosy germs grown in the laboratory are very different from the typical acid-fast rods that are seen in the diseased leprosy tissue. Eleanor explained that cultured leprosy microbes are similar to unusual growth forms of bacteria that microbiologists have termed "L" forms, or "pleuropneumonia-like organisms" (PPLO), or "cell wall deficient bacteria."

Fourteen years later, in 1965, in the same *Journal of Leprosy*, B.R. Chaterjee also succeeded in culturing the leprosy microbe ("Growth habits of *Mycobacterium lepra*") [13]. Chatterjee's leprosy microbe also existed in a variety of forms, only one of which was the acid-fast rod. Neither Chatterjee nor *The Journal* mentioned Eleanor's previous success in growing similar leprosy microbes.

Despite these reports, medical and microbiology textbooks still state the century-old dogma that the microbe of leprosy has never been grown in culture. And the leprosy research of Alexander-Jackson, Chatterjee, and others, is never mentioned.

Why does the scientific community ignore important research which could lead to better treatment methods and a possible cure for leprosy? Is it because of scientific ignorance, or is it a deliberate attempt by the international leprosy establishment to deceive and maintain the status quo in leprosy treatment and research? Perhaps future medical historians will provide satisfactory answers to these questions.

While Eleanor was busy at Cornell, Virginia was seeking financial support to open a laboratory for cancer microbe research. Grants were obtained from The American Cancer Society, The Damon Runyon Fund, Abbott Laboratories, and others. On June 2, 1949, the laboratory opened at the Presbyterian Hospital in Newark, New Jersey. Virginia was made director.

The years 1949-1953 were highly productive for cancer microbe research. Eleanor carefully pondered whether to leave Cornell and join the Newark lab. Finally, the lure of working with the cancer microbe was overwhelming. In 1951 Eleanor began commuting from her Manhattan apartment to Newark. They were the happiest years of her life.

Virginia knew how to detect the hidden killer in cancer. The key was the acid-fast stain which made the hidden cancer microbe visible. Eleanor knew every guise of the microbe, and how it survived and multipied inside the body. The two women were determined to prove that the cancer microbe caused cancer.

Shortly after the lab opened, Virginia read an article in *Life* magazine about Irene Diller Ph.D., a researcher in the Department of Chemotherapy at the Institute for Cancer Research in Philadelphia. Irene was an expert

cytologist, a "cell" specialist who studied the effects of
anti-cancer drugs on cancer cells in animals. One day
she noticed a peculiar fungus-like filament sticking out
of a cancer cell. She then observed the same phenomenon
in other types of cancer cells. Irene began to culture
cancer tumors and grew strange-looking microbes. She
reported these microbiologic findings at a meeting of the
American Association for the Advancement of Science;
and *Time* and *Life* magazine picked up the story.

Virginia and Eleanor met Irene and told her about the
cancer microbe and its fungal forms, and how the acid-
fast stain was the key to its identification. Virginia,
Eleanor, and Irene formed a professional association
which lasted until Irene's death in 1988, at age 88.
Eleanor affectionately termed their trio "The Three
Musketeers" of cancer research.

Irene's specialty was experimenting with mice and rats
who were genetically inbred for cancer research. After
learning about the cancer microbe, she began testing
thousands of animals for cancer microbe infection. By
injecting young male albino mice with cancer microbes
she doubled the rate of cancer in the mice.

The Three Musketeers proved "Koch's postulates"
with the cancer microbe. The microbe was cultured from
cancer tumors and from the blood. When injected into
animals it produced cancer; and the cancer microbe was
recultured from the tumors of the animals [14-15].

The animal experiments proved that the cancer
microbe caused cancer. Virginia and Eleanor envisioned
a vaccine that could be used against the cancer microbe.
They began experiments to test a vaccine. The trio was
closing in on the biggest medical mystery of the
twentieth century, and powerful people in the cancer
establishment were taking careful note of their research.

The three women were headed for big trouble.

Nineteen fifty-three was a momentous year for Virginia and Eleanor. In June the Newark lab team presented their cancer research at an exhibit at the American Medical Association meeting, held at the Waldorf-Astoria Hotel in New York City. RCA generously lent an electron microscope which televised the "live" cancer microbe to the audience. Roy Allen's beautiful color microphotographs and James Hillier's spectacular electron microscopic photos were the hit of the AMA convention.

Immediately, the dark forces went into action against the women. According to Virginia's autobiography (*CANCER: A NEW BREAKTHROUGH*), Virginia and Eleanor had made enemies at the highest echelons of cancer research. The big boys in the medical establishment knew the identification of a cancer microbe could destroy millions of dollars worth of cancer research. The microbe and its implications were a serious threat to the pharmaceutical industry and the cancer research establishment. The discovery of an infectious agent in cancer would rock the scientific world and threaten the multi-billion cancer treatment industry. A "cause" and a vaccine "cure" for cancer would be financially disastrous for the biomedical business world.

Virginia believes that Cornelius Rhodes, head of Sloan-Kettering Memorial Hospital, was the powerful man that destroyed her dream. His financial interests would be ruined by her cancer discoveries. Virginia insists Rhoades put pressure on the press to kill the cancer microbe story. As a result, there was a press black-out of the exhibit at the AMA convention.

In September, Virginia and Eleanor presented papers at the Sixth International Conference for Microbiology

in Rome. The conference was a great success and the
two women met other European scientists, who had also
studied the cancer microbe.

While Virginia and Eleanor vacationed in Europe,
their enemies succeeded in pulling grant money away
from the Newark lab, forcing its closure. Without money,
there could be no cancer microbe research. And without
research the new cancer breakthrough would die a
natural death.

Disheartened, disillusioned, and totally defeated,
Virginia moved to California. Eleanor got a job with a
private firm. Things were never quite the same again,
although the two women were hardly finished. In the
1960s, Eleanor secured a grant from the National
Institutes of Health to study the Rous sarcoma virus, a
virus that causes sarcoma cancer in chickens. Eleanor
proved the Rous virus is actually a filterable form of the
cancer microbe. Using cancer bacteria cultured from
Rous virus-infected chicken sarcoma tumors, Eleanor
made an anti-cancer tumor vaccine. Amazingly, her
vaccine protected healthy chickens against Rous sarcoma
disease! As usual, Eleanor's research was ignored
because none of the virologists wanted to believe that the
Rous virus originated from a bacterium[16-17].

In the 1960s another distinguished woman scientist
joined the cancer microbe trio. Florence Seibert (1897-)
is one of the most respected names in biochemistry. Her
most notable achievement was the development of a skin
diagnostic test for TB — the so-called PPD (purified
protein derivative) skin test. In 1938 she was awarded
the highest honor in TB research, the Trudeau Medal
given by the National Tuberculosis Association.

Florence learned about the cancer microbe through

Irene Diller. Astounded by its similarity to the tubercle bacillus, Florence developed a keen interest in the microbiology of cancer. She retired to Florida in 1958 but the compulsion to study the cancer microbe finally forced her out of retirement in 1964.

In her autobiography, *PEBBLES ON THE HILL OF A SCIENTIST* (1968)[18] published privately in St. Petersburg, she wrote about her experiences with the microbe. "We found that we were able to isolate bacteria from every piece of tumor and every acute leukemic blood specimen that we had. They are a strange breed of bacteria. . . they seem to have some properties like the mycobacteria (to which the tubercle bacillus belongs); like the corynebacteria (to which the diphtheria bacillus belongs); and like the well known staphylococcus or micrococcus. But they are not wholly like any of these, and so we think they are a group of their own, bordering on these other forms."

Florence was also surprised by the diversity of forms of the cancer microbe. "One of the most interesting properties of these bacteria is their great pleomorphism. For example, they readily change their shape from round cocci to elongated rods, and even to long thread-like filaments depending upon what medium they grow on and how long they grow. . . And even more interesting than this is the fact that these bacteria have a filterable form in their life cycle; that is, they can become so small that they pass through bacterial filters which hold back bacteria. This (ability to pass through bacterial filters) is what viruses do, and is one of the main criteria of a virus, separating them from bacteria. But the viruses also will not live on artificial media like these bacteria do. They need body tissue to grow on. Our filterable form, however, can be recovered again on ordinary

artificial bacterial media and will grow on these. This
should interest the virus workers very much and should
cause them to ask themselves how many of their viruses
may not be filterable forms of our bacteria."[18]

In 1969 the cancer microbiologists were finally given an
opportunity to speak at a conference entitled "Unusual
Isolates From Clinical Material." The meeting, sponsored
by the New York Academy of Sciences, was held at the
Waldorf Astoria. Virginia, Eleanor, Irene, Florence, and
a host of other microbiologists all spoke about their
experiences with the cancer microbe. The proceedings of
the conference are officially recorded in the *Annals of
the New York Academy of Science* (Volume 174; 1970).
This Volume is an indispensable document for students
of the cancer microbe.
  Despite brilliant presentations at the conference,
nothing changed. The leading physicians in medical
science simply refused to recognize the reality of the
cancer microbe; and those who championed the microbe
were still considered oddballs.
  There are dozens of scientists who have studied the
cancer microbe, and Virginia always gave credit to them
in her writings. And yet, not a single one of them has
received recognition for the most important medical
discovery of this century.
  Cancer microbe research is a jinx — a one-way ticket
to scientific oblivion. The medical community is supposedly committed to finding the "cause" of cancer. But
this is a myth. In truth the medical establishment is
quick to squelch anyone who proposes either a cause or
a cure for cancer. Most physicians will deny this, but I
know it is the truth because I have studied the history of
the cancer microbe.

The history of the cancer microbe is indeed a sad commentary on "modern" medical science and its leadership.

References:

1. **Alexander-Jackson E**: Differential triple stain for demonstrating and studying non-acid-fast forms of the tubercle bacillus in sputum, tissue and body fluids. Science 99: 307-308, 1944.

2. **Much H**: Die nach Ziehl nicht darstellbaren Formen des Tuberkelbacillus. Berlin Klin Wochenschr 45: 691-694, 1908.

3. **Fontes A**: Uber die Filtrierbarkeit des Tuberkelvirus vom Standpunkte des Polymorphismus. Beitr Klin Tuberk 77: 1-15, 1931.

4. **Alexander-Jackson A**: A hitherto undemonstrated zoogleal form of *Mycobacterium tuberculosis*. Ann NY Acad Sci 46: 127-152, 1945.

5. **Sweany HC**: The granules of the tubercle bacillus. Amer Rev Tuberc 17: 53-76, 1928.

6. **Sweany HC**: The filterability of the tubercle bacillus. Amer Rev Tuberc 17: 77-85, 1928.

7. **Sweany HC**: Mutation forms of the tubercle bacilus. JAMA 87: 1206-1211, 1928.

8. **Pla y Armengol R**: Die verschiedenen Formen des Tuberkuloserregers. Beitr Klin Tuberk 77: 47-55, 1931.

9. **Mellon RR and Fisher LW**: New studies on the filterability of pure cultures of the tubercle group of micro-organisms. J Infect Dis 51: 117-128, 1932.

10. **Mellon RR and Beinhauer LG**: The pathogenesis of noncaseating tuberculosis of the skin and lymph glands. Arch Dermatol Syph 36: 515-533, 1937.

11. **Beinhauer LG and Mellon RR**: Pathogenesis of noncaseating epithelioid tuberculosis of hypoderm and lymph glands. Arch Dermatol Syph 37: 451-460, 1938.

12. **Alexander-Jackson E**: The cultivation and morphological study of a pleomorphic organism from the blood of leprosy patients. Intl J Leprosy 19: 173-186, 1951.

13. **Chatterjee BR**: Growth habits of *Mycobacterium leprae*. Intl J Leprosy 33: 551-562, 1965.

14. **Diller IC**: Tumor incidence in ICR/Albino and C57/B16JNIcr male mice injected with organisms cultured from mouse malignant tissues. Growth 38: 505-517, 1974.

15. **Diller IC and Donnelly AJ**: Experiments with mammalian tumor isolates. Ann NY Acad Sci 174: 655-674, 1970.

16. **Alexander-Jackson E**: Ultraviolet spectrogramic microscope studies of Rous sarcoma virus cultured in cell-free medium. Ann NY Acad Sci 174: 765-781, 1970.

17. **Alexander-Jackson E**: Mycoplasma (PPLO) isolated from Rous sarcoma virus. Growth 30: 199-228, 1966.

18. **Seibert FB**: *Pebbles on the Hill of a Scientist*. St. Petersburg, Florida, 1968.

CHAPTER SEVEN

The Sarcoidosis Connection

While Virginia, Eleanor, Irene, and Florence were telling the medical world about the cancer microbe, I was content to study scleroderma. I was sure dermatologists and pathologists would soon confirm my finding of acid-fast bacteria in this disease.

Hunting for acid-fast rods in scleroderma tissue was as frustrating as looking for four-leaf clovers. Nevertheless, Dan Kelso and I were determined to keep the scleroderma research alive. We were rewarded when the *Archives of Dermatology* published our scleroderma findings in 1971[1]. We cited Virginia's original discovery of the scleroderma microbe in 1947 and the confirmation of her work by scientists at the Pasteur Institute in Brussels in 1953[2]. We also wrote about the allied cancer microbe research undertaken by Virginia, Eleanor Alexander-Jackson, Irene Diller and Florence Seibert.

Now that my scleroderma research was published in the world's most prestigious dermatology journal, I was content to sit on my laurels. I had no intention of being a medical researcher and I wanted to get on with my personal life.

Virginia kept prodding me to get involved in the cancer microbe but her research was too controversial. The American Cancer Society (ACS) had already blasted Virginia and Eleanor for their proposed treatment of cancer, which consisted of antibiotics, diet and megavitamin therapy, and an anti-cancer vaccine made from killed cultures of the patient's own cancer microbe.

At the 1966 ACS Science Writer's Seminar, Virginia and Eleanor angered officials by reporting that their proposed cancer treatment appeared to make the cancer process "reversible." Dr. Jorgen Fogh, a spokesman for the ACS and a virologist at Sloan-Kettering Institute for Cancer Research in New York City, claimed he had examined over 150 human cancers and had never found the cancer microbe. The ACS did readily concede that various microbes could be isolated from cancer patients because they are so susceptible to infection. However, the Society insisted these microbes were not connected with the cause of cancer.

The ACS issued a "statement" against Virginia's anti-cancer vaccine to 58 Divisions of the organization, which was subsequently published in January 1968 in the Society's official publication (Unproven Methods of Cancer Treatment: The Livingston Vaccine, *CA—A Cancer Journal for Clinicians*, Volume 18, pp 46-47). The ACS concluded there was no evidence to incriminate bacteria in any form of cancer.

There was no way I wanted to get involved in Virginia's feud with the cancer establishment.

———

In 1967 my parents moved to Palm Springs, a two-hour drive from Hollywood. Because of my homosexuality, I had wanted to live my life far away from my parents' view. Now they were living close by.

Although he never told me, I later discovered that my father was never happy about my decision to study dermatology. Before his illness, he secretly hoped I would become an orthopedic surgeon, and he envisioned a practice where he would work side by side with his two surgeon sons. My brother Howard told me that when Dad first learned of my decision to be a dermatologist, he expressed his disappointment and disdain by declaring, "I can't believe my son would want to be a cosmetician!" Nevertheless, he seemed proud of my published scleroderma research, even though he understood little about it.

Dad was overjoyed when Howard chose to study orthopedic surgery. But by this time he realized his fantasy of practising with his surgeon son could never be fulfilled. He was unable to walk, to speak clearly, to cut his food, or even lift himself out of a chair without assistance. For hours he stared out the window of his small mobile home in Palm Springs, mulling over his plight and his abandonment by the medical profession he had so dearly loved.

While my father was living out the last years of his life, I was busy enjoying my life as a physician. In 1969 I finally found Mr. Right in the form of a tall and handsome dancer. We moved into a new home and furnished it with all the proper decorator touches. And for a few years we were happy.

With my busy professional and social life, there was little time for medical research. After five years, my relationship with Mr. Right became unbearable and ended disastrously when we became physically violent toward each other. When a handgun was brought into the house, I feared for my life. My love affair turned into a gay soap opera of the worst sort.

When I finally freed myself from this intolerable situation in 1974, I was emotionally and financially devastated. That same year Father died of his disease, and Mother decided to remain in Palm Springs. She had nursed Father for over a decade and she missed him terribly. My sister had married and moved back east; and Howard was serving as a physician in the Navy. After his tour of duty, he moved his family out to California and settled in nearby Pasadena.

I had given up on finding love, but shortly after my breakup I met Frank — a short, energetic, dark-eyed Italian who instantly reminded me of half the Italian cousins I grew up with. He possessed all the intellectual abilities I lacked. With ease he could fix a flat, repair a leaking toilet, rewire a lamp, replace a garbage disposal — and he cooked the best lasagna I ever tasted.

Frank showered me with affection and made me feel happy and secure; but I had always been unlucky in love and I hesitated to enter another relationship. It had taken several years to get over the loss of my first lover, Bob. And my second relationship nearly destroyed me.

I had never met anyone quite like Frank. With time I grew more and more fond of him. There was no way I could let him out of my life, even if the timing for another love affair seemed inappropriate. Throwing caution to the wind, I entered the most intense relationship of my life. It was a wise decision. We have been together for fifteen years and we remain each other's best friend. There is a spiritual bond between us that can never be broken, no matter what.

My first lover, Bob, still holds a special place in my memories. After our breakup in 1962, I occasionally saw him at the beach. He remained remarkably handsome and trim, even though I suspected he drank and smoked too much. After me, he had a steady stream of white, black, Latin, and Asian lovers. His romances usually lasted a few months until he tired of them and moved on to another.

The last time I saw him was at a gay bar in the summer of 1975. I introduced him to Frank, and Bob introduced us to his new black lover. We chatted a while and parted. I can't recall anything special that was said, just the usual bar talk. But I was genuinely glad to see Bob. For the first time, I felt no resentment toward him for breaking my heart. I was happy with Frank; and Bob seemed content with his new friend.

A year later, Frank and I were attending a Hollywood Bowl concert. Rick Hernandez spotted us and came over to say hello. "Did you hear about Bob?" he asked. "What do you mean?" I answered.

"He was killed in a freeway accident last winter. It was late at night. He and his black friend were out drinking and Bob crashed into the back of a huge truck. The car was totally wrecked. His friend was asleep in the front seat. It's a miracle he came out alive!"

As the floodlights dimmed and the starlight concert began, images of Bob flooded my brain. I had always envied his romantic adventures, and now he was dead and I would never see him again. Fourteen years earlier when I first fell madly in love with him, he was a young man of twenty-four and I was twenty-eight. Bob would have hated getting old. Losing his good looks and his lean body would have devastated him. I wondered if he lived his life so adventurously because he knew he would die young. Despite all the heartbreak, I was glad he came into my life and briefly shared his magic brand of love.

It was comforting having Frank at my side. He brought a peacefulness and a stability to my life that I greatly needed, and once again I was able to think clearly.

And now that I was content I knew the time was drawing closer for me to get back into my medical studies with those little red bugs that fascinated me so.

———

I met Abe Greenstein in January 1977. He was referred to me because he had a very rare type of scleroderma known as "nodular scleroderma." Instead of having large areas of skin hardening, Abe's scleroderma consisted of hard bumps of skin with "normal" skin in between. No dermatologist in the city had ever seen a case like Abe's; and only a handful of "nodular scleroderma" cases were recorded in the medical literature.

As Abe undressed, he said, "My dermatologist tells me you have studied scleroderma. He says you know what causes it."

I explained that I had found TB germs in scleroderma but that I didn't know how to cure it. Abe told me his parents had TB when he was a young boy.

"Are you still doing research?" he asked.

"I haven't studied any new scleroderma cases in a long time," I admitted.

Looking into my eyes, Abe said, "Why did you stop doing research?"

His question struck like lightning. I thought of reasons why I had put aside my research, but none of them were valid. I possessed a special research talent and I wasn't using it. Abe's stare was unrelenting and the brief moment seemed like an eternity. I felt locked into a strange mystical experience that was urging me back into research.

Finally Abe's searing eyes turned away. "I want you to study my case," he said firmly. " I will do anything you want me to do."

From that moment my scleroderma research resumed with a frenzy. Miraculously, I easily found acid-fast rods in Abe's skin tissue. He urged me to take as many skin biopsy samples as I needed. I was disappointed when Dan Kelso repeatedly cultured pleomorphic microbes that looked like common staphylococci and common coccobacilli (corynebacteria). Where were the acid-fast rods? Finally, on one smear of a 13-day culture we identified acid-fast bacteria that looked exactly like typical TB microbes! Abe's unusual scleroderma case and microbiological findings were published in the *Archives of Dermatology* in 1980.

After studying scleroderma tissue for over ten years, I began to pay attention to the tissue "granules" that I had previously ignored. Virginia and Eleanor claimed the granules were actual forms of the scleroderma microbe; but the expert pathologists and dermatologists insisted the granules were "mast cell granules." (Mast cells are common tissue cells filled with granules.) How could I ever convince these specialists that the "granules" were microbes?

I simply could not believe that every "granule" I saw in scleroderma was a mast cell granule. I argued that if the "granules" originated from mast cells it was necessary to see the "nucleus" of the mast cell. In the scattered and clumped collections of granules, there was frequently no nucleus that I could detect. But the pathologists claimed that it wasn't necessary to identify a nucleus in order to identify mast cell granules. Of course, the pathologists paid no attention to the "granular" microbes that we cultured from scleroderma. Some of these scleroderma microbes were the exact size and shape of the granules in the scleroderma tissue. I stopped paying attention to the pathologists. I convinced myself that at least "some" of the "granules" were microbes.

Eleanor kept reassuring me the granules were not mast cell granules. In Eleanor's opinion, the granules represented the tiny round coccoid forms of the pleomorphic scleroderma microbe. But how could I prove this to pathologists and dermatologists who knew nothing about scleroderma microbes? Eleanor said the granules were "cell-wall deficient forms," but I knew nothing about such things. Finally, in desperation, Eleanor said, "Alan, you really must read Professor Lida Mattman's book. She teaches microbiology at Wayne State University in Detroit, and she explains it all clearly."

When I read Lida Mattman's *CELL WALL DEFI- CIENT FORMS* (1974)[4] I was stunned. I learned that bacteria, especially tuberculosis-type microbes, exist in many different forms! Lida and her colleagues proved that TB microbes have a cycle of growth that encom- passes many different "cell wall deficient forms," such as virus-size forms, bacterial forms, and giant forms known as "large bodies." Amazingly, the tubercle bacillus and other bacteria can grow into "large body" structures, which can attain the size of red blood cells, or even larger[5]! (I was later able to detect "large bodies" in cancer, AIDS, and other diseases.) According to Lida, "Much's granules" and Eleanor's "zooglear" forms are also part of the life cycle of TB microbes.

The various forms and sizes and shapes of the TB microbe are all the result of changes in the "cell wall" of the microbe. After studying Lida's book, I concluded that the granular and round coccoid forms of the scleroderma microbe had the characteristics of Lida's so-

called "cell wall deficient forms." The editors of the
Archives of Dermatology kindly allowed me to present
these revolutionary ideas in our paper describing Abe's
"nodular scleroderma."[3] The knowledge I gained from
Lida Mattman proved invaluable in my scleroderma and
cancer research.

Florence Seibert offered valuable advice and encouragement in her letters. She advised me to study
autopsied cases of scleroderma. If I could demonstrate
the scleroderma microbe in the internal organs, Florence
was sure I could convince pathologists that the scleroderma germ existed. But how could I study autopsies? I
was a dermatologist, not a pathologist!

With the help of a pathologist I learned how to study
autopsy tissue. I chose Hilda Sanchez as my first
autopsy case. Hilda died of scleroderma in 1969. Before
her death I discovered a few, typical acid-fast bacteria in
her skin tissue sections, and Dan cultured pleomorphic
microbes from her skin biopsies.

The pathologist sent me a shoe box containing forty
pieces of Hilda's scleroderma tissue permanently "fixed"
and embedded in small blocks of paraffin wax. We
numbered each paraffin block before cutting the tissue
into sections. The numbered sections of tissue were
placed onto glass slides each marked with a correspond-
ing number. After the tissue was stained with an acid-
fast stain, the pathologist recorded the exact organs and
tissue mounted on each numbered slide. The system
worked perfectly. In this way I was later able to look for
the cancer microbe in autopsied patients who died of
cancer and AIDS.

In acid-fast stained sections of Hilda's heart, lungs,
kidneys, adrenal glands, and connective tissue, I
discovered the same-appearing pleomorphic bacteria that

I had seen in her sclerodermatous skin. There was no doubt that these scleroderma microbes had killed her. In 1980 *Dermatologica* published Hilda's autopsy study, which included eight photos showing her scleroderma germ in culture, and in her internal organs[6].

Fifteen years earlier I had first seen acid-fast bacteria in Reuben's scleroderma. I had anticipated that some other dermatologist or pathologist would surely see or culture the scleroderma microbe in other cases and confirm my work. But as the years passed there was no confirmation, and my research papers were never cited in articles on scleroderma. Thus, the idea of a scleroderma microbe quickly vanished from the medical literature.

————

The years after Father's death in 1974 were lonely ones for Mother. Frank and I tried to cheer her up when she came for visits. I wanted her to know that Frank was more than just my best friend, and I was tired of pretending to be straight when I wasn't. In the mid-1970s, gays were organizing to fight the political forces that sought to limit the civil rights of homosexuals. It was time for me to come out of the closet, march in the Gay Pride parade, and be honest with Mother for the first time in my life.

I finally got up the courage to speak with her. "Mother, there is something I must tell you. It's been on my mind for a long time and I hope you won't be too upset, but I want you to know that I am a homosexual. And Frank is more that just a friend, he's my lover. Now that you and I are spending so much time together, I can't hide it any longer." I took a deep breath and anxiously awaited her response.

Mother was silent for a few moments, and then answered calmly. "Years ago your father told me you were homosexual. I really am very sorry you're that way. But I don't think your father and I did anything wrong. We always tried to do the right thing."

"But if Dad knew, why didn't he ever say anything to me?" I implored.

"He figured you didn't want to talk about it. You never really did, you know."

She continued. "You're my son and I love you very much. But I don't understand two men getting together. Your father was the only man I ever loved. He was the only man I ever knew. Even with his disease, and even though he had no strength in his arms and legs, he still wanted me to make love to him. It was very difficult, but I did it because I loved him. I wish to God I could have him back with me, sickness and all. He was my whole life and now there's very little left for me. But I'm sorry, I just don't understand two men together. I don't."

I never discussed my gay life with Mother again. She seemed uncomfortable with the subject; and she went about as if nothing had changed. I'm sure she would never have chosen to have a gay son, but that was her destiny. In 1979 she travelled with Howard's family to Paris and London. They sailed back to New York on the Queen Elizabeth II. She was marvelously happy for the first time in years. A few days later, she died suddenly of a massive heart attack. After Dad had passed away, Mom always prayed for a quick death because she dreaded the thought of being a burden to anyone. She was a good woman, and I'm glad her prayers were heard.

The Gay Pride movement reached its apex in the late 1970s. Trendy homosexual ghettos sprang up in Manhattan, West Hollywood and San Francisco. Bars, discos, and homosexual businesses flourished in the new sexual climate. For an entry fee of a few dollars, gay bathhouses offered an unlimited supply of men and erotic adventures. Marijuana and designer drugs were commonplace, and it was suddenly fashionable to be gay. Not since the days of the Roman Empire had anyone seen the likes of the new bacchanal.

The health risks of the new sexual freedom were few. Perhaps a case of gonorrhea or syphilis, both curable with antibiotics. At worst, hepatitis and herpes. Nothing could stop the gay party: not Anita Bryant and the right-wing antigay conservatives; not the admonitions of the pope and the religious leaders; and not the government health officials who were appalled at the sexually-transmitted disease statistics among male homosexuals.

Many homosexuals and heterosexuals complained it was hard to find love and romance in the new sexual milieu, but with the unending supply of sex, who cared about love and commitment? By the end of the seventies the party was winding down, but few people noticed.

In 1978, a strange virus of unknown origin began appearing in the gay ghettos of Manhattan, West Hollywood and San Francisco. Within a few years, the virus transformed the gay love-in into a death watch of unprecedented proportions. The most promiscuous, the kinkiest, the most drug-addicted, and the best-looking men would be the first to die.

It took another half-decade to recognize the severity of the holocaust that was decimating the gay communities in America. In the mid-1980s, government epidemiologists predicted that half the men living in the gay ghettos would be dead by the 1990s.

The prediction was probably accurate. By 1989, fifty percent of gay men living in San Francisco were believed to be infected with the AIDS virus.

———

At the dermatology clinic in 1977, Lyon Rowe MD and I encountered two women with an unusual form of "pseudoscleroderma" of the legs. Although the skin of the leg was hardened like scleroderma, these women did not have typical scleroderma. I discovered acid-fast microbes and "large bodies" in the diseased skin of these two women, and our findings were reported in the *Archives of Dermatology* in 1979.[7]

I also studied Georgette, another woman with pseudoscleroderma who also had "sarcoidosis." Sarcoidosis is a disease that can affect many organs of the body. Most commonly, the disease affects the lungs. Lung sarcoidosis can closely resemble TB. It is generally agreed that there are no microbes in sarcoidosis, and the disease is another "disease of unknown etiology."

I biopsied the hard skin of Georgette's leg and was amazed by the pathologist's diagnostic report. Her skin showed the usual scleroderma changes, but it also showed "sarcoidosis." I had never seen scleroderma tissue "mixed" with the pathologic changes of sarcoidosis.

Georgette was born in 1924. In the early 1970s her eyes became severely inflamed due to "uveitis," and she went blind. In 1975 a surgeon removed one of her lungs and some lymph nodes because of suspected lung cancer. After the tissue was examined, the pathologist discovered that Georgette had lung sarcoidosis, not cancer. Because sarcoidosis tissue can resemble tuberculosis, the laboratory tested the lung tissue for TB microbes. None was found. Georgette's doctors finally agreed that her uveitis and blindness were related to her sarcoidosis diagnosis.

Several other biopsies of Georgette's leg lesions all showed scleroderma-like changes. The scleroderma microbe was detected in her tissue; and Dan cultured *Staphylococcus epidermidis* from her diseased skin. Some of the cultured staphylococci were acid-fast. I requested stored samples of Georgette's lung and lymph node tissue, and stained them with Lida Mattman's stain. Microbes were detected in all the sarcoidosis specimens. Georgette's interesting case of pseudoscleroderma and sarcoidosis was reported in *Dermatologica* in 1981[8].

While studying Georgette's tissue, I also checked the tissue of two other patients with sarcoid skin lesions, and one patient with sarcoidosis of the lymph nodes. All this sarcoid tissue showed pleomorphic bacteria! Dan was able to culture a pleomorphic, coccobacillary microbe (*Propionibacterium acnes*) from one skin sarcoid case; the other case was "negative." In 1982 *Growth* published a paper showing photos of the sarcoid microbes detected in these three cases[9].

Sarcoidosis was discovered a century ago. Since that time, dozens of scientists have observed microbes in sarcoid tissue, and pleomorphic bacteria have been cultured. Details of these sarcoid microbes can be found in papers by Crawford[10], Gullberg[11], Beinhauer and Mellon[12], Schaumann and Hallberg[13, 14], Mitsuoka et al[15], and other researchers.

Dr. C. Xalabarder of the Francisco Moragas Antituberculosis Institute in Barcelona, Spain, experimentally produced sarcoidosis in animals by injecting them with cell wall deficient forms of TB microbes that he cultured from "inactive" TB cases[16]. On the basis of his extensive research Dr. Xalabarder concluded that sarcoidosis is a form of tuberculosis caused by pleomorphic TB germs. *He also produced cancerous tissue changes in animals by injecting them with pleomorphic TB microbes!*[16]. Despite all this research showing microbes in sarcoidosis, it is still taught in medical school that there are no microbes in this disease!

For many years scientists have recognized a peculiar relationship between sarcoidosis and cancer (especially lymphoma cancer). For example, pathologists occasionally encounter sarcoidosis tissue changes in lymph nodes which drain cancer tissue. One of my elderly patients with skin lesions of sarcoid had no signs of lung sarcoidosis or cancer. However, a year later she began to experience night sweats, fever and chills, and swelling of her lymph nodes. One of these enlarged neck nodes was removed and the pathologist found lymphoma cancer. Photographs of the acid-fast microbes I discovered in her skin sarcoid lesions and in the cancerous lymph nodes were published in the *International Journal of Dermatology* in 1982[17].

Although microbes are not recognized in sarcoidosis, I detected pleomorphic microbes in all my sarcoidosis patients. Unfortunately, most pathologists are trained to detect only the "classic" acid-fast rod form of the tubercle bacillus. Thus, pleomorphic forms of TB bacteria are not recognized and go undetected.

For this reason, the cause of sarcoidosis remains unknown, and the sarcoid microbe is only rarely mentioned in the scientific literature. This is a tragedy for Georgette and thousands of other sarcoidosis sufferers who are infected with microbes unrecognized by medical science. Even more tragic are the millions of cancer patients, who are infected with deadly cancer microbes that are ignored by cancer experts.

After I had studied the strange link between sarcoidosis and cancer, it was inevitable that I would begin to study cancer. For years I put off studying cancer because I didn't want to be controversial like Virginia. But as I grew wiser in the ways of medical science, I realized I had the special knowledge and talent to study the cancer microbe.

The die was cast when a young mother with four children sought my advice about some small lumps which had recently appeared on her chest. When Alice undressed I saw the scars on her chest and the absence of breasts. I took a skin biopsy for the pathologist and sent an additional specimen to Dan Kelso for culture.

I had seen the cancer microbe in lymphoma and in sarcoidosis. Soon I would see the same microbe in this young mother's metastatic breast cancer. I knew that all the cancer experts in the world didn't have the foggiest idea how to save Alice's life.

I was forty-five years old and I was beginnning to understand my purpose in life, and why I was "different" from the rest. I knew I had the God-given power and the courage to join Virginia in showing the cancer microbe to the world. I could no longer remain silent.

And I no longer gave a damn about the consequences.

References:

1. **Cantwell AR Jr, Kelso DW**: Acid-fast bacteria in scleroderma and morphea. Arch Dermatol 104: 21-

25, 1971.

2. **Delmotte N, van der Meiren L**: Recherches bacteriologiques et histologiques concernant la sclerodermie. Dermatologica 107: 177-182, 1953.

3. **Cantwell AR Jr, Kelso DW**: Nodular scleroderma and pleomorphic acid-fast bacteria. Arch Dermatol 116: 1283-1290. 1980.

4. **Mattman LH**: *Cell Wall Deficient Forms.* CRC Press, Cleveland, Ohio, 1974.

5. **Mattman LH, Tinstall LH, Mathews WW, et al**: L variation in mycobacteria. Am Rev Respir Dis 82: 202-211, 1960.

6. **Cantwell AR Jr, Kelso DW**: Autopsy findings of nonacid-fast bacteria in scleroderma. Dermatologica 160: 90-99, 1980.

7. **Cantwell AR Jr, Kelso DW**: Hypodermitis sclerodermiformis and unusual acid-fast bacteria. Arch Dermatol 115: 449-452, 1979.

8. **Cantwell AR Jr**: Variably acid-fast bacteria in a case of systemic sarcoidosis and hypodermitis sclerodermiformis. Dermatologica 163: 239-248, 1981.

9. **Cantwell AR Jr**: Histologic observations of variably acid-fast bacteria in systemic sarcoidosis: A report of three cases. Growth 46: 113-125, 1982.

10. **Crawford S**: Cutaneous nodulodiscoid tuberculosis of anergic type. Arch Dermatol Syph 27: 755-777, 1933.

11. **Gullberg E**: Some observations indicating the

possibility of a relation of the bacillus of Koch to a yeast-like fungus (of odium type). Acta Med Scand 94: 527-566, 1938.

12. **Beinhauer LG, Mellon RR**: Pathogenesis of noncaseating epithelioid tuberculosis of hypoderm and lymph glands. Arch Dermatol Syph 37: 451-460, 1938.

13. **Schaumann J**: On the nature of certain peculiar corpuscles present in the tissue of lymphogranulomatosis benigna. Acta Med Scandinav 106: 239-253, 1941.

14. **Schaumann J, Hallberg V**: Koch's bacilli manifested in the tissue of lymphogranulomatosis benigna (Schaumann) by using Hallberg's staining method. Acta Med Scandinav 107: 499-501, 1941.

15. **Mitsuoka TY, Benno Y, Homma JY, et al**: Characterization of *Propionibacterium acnes* isolated form patients with sarcoidosis. Japan J Exp Med 48: 275-277, 1978.

16. **Xalabarder C**: Sarcoidosis experimental. Publ Inst Antituberc (Barcelona) 18: 51-76, 1969.

17. **Cantwell AR Jr**: Variably acid-fast bacteria in a rare case of coexistent malignant lymphoma and cutaneous sarcoid-like granulomas. Intl J Dermatol 21: 99-106, 1982.

CHAPTER EIGHT

The Cancer Microbe

Alice's skin biopsy report confirmed that the breast cancer had returned. The spread of her cancer to the skin meant that her prognosis was dismal. I arranged to have Alice's tissue sections specially colored with Lida Mattman's acid-fast stain. When I carefully examined the cancerous tissue, the acid-fast coccoid forms of the cancer microbe were visible. I checked the tissue of three other women whose breast cancer had spread to the skin. All three showed the microbe.

Dan Kelso cultured *Staphylococcus epidermidis* from Alice's cancerous skin. As the culture aged, the cocci transformed into larger globoids and rods and yeast-like forms; and acid-fast granules were abundant.

I examined acid-fast stained sections of Alice's original breast tumor that had been removed a year earlier. The microbe was present in the breast tumor. The microbe was also present in the breast tissue that the pathologist had labelled "normal" and cancer-free. This indicated the cancer microbe existed in the cancer-free tissue *before* the tissue became cancerous!

Unfortunately, when Alice's breast cancer was removed, it had already spread to the lymph nodes. Shortly after I examined Alice, the cancer also spread to her lungs and liver. She died several months later. Photographs of the microbes in Alice's breast cancer tumor, and pictures of the cancer microbe Dan cultured were published in our article on the microbiology of breast cancer, which appeared in *The Journal of*

Dermatologic Surgery and Oncology in 1981[1].

Now that I knew how to detect the acid-fast cancer microbe in tissue sections, I studied Hodgkin's disease (a special form of lymphoma); mycosis fungoides (a rare form of skin lymphoma); and Kaposi's sarcoma (a rare form of skin cancer). A few years later, Kaposi's sarcoma became well-known as the so-called "gay cancer" in homosexual men with AIDS. The cancer microbe was present in the skin tumors of all these three different kinds of cancer; and Dan Kelso was successful in growing staphylococci and coccobacilli from the cancerous tissue. Some of the pleomorphic microbes were acid-fast.

I knew doctors would be highly skeptical about these microbes because the cancer microbes we cultured were similar to common skin germs. In order to show that these microbes were killing cancer patients, I followed Florence Seibert's advice and studied autopsy cases of lymphoma, Hodgkin's disease, mycosis fungoides, and Kaposi's sarcoma. Using the acid-fast stain I discovered the cancer microbe in the diseased tissue of patients who died of these cancers. My microbiologic and histologic studies of these four different cancers were published in peer-reviewed medical journals[2-5].

All this research proved the cancer microbe is a reality. The cell wall deficient cancer microbe is *always* present in cancer and its forms are varied: cocci, rods, large globoid and yeast-like forms, acid-fast granules, fungus-like forms, and giant "large body" forms. Because most physicians are taught little about cell wall deficient bacteria, the cancer microbe remains the hidden killer in cancer.

Against all odds I had become a microbe hunter like the nineteenth century medical scientists I had read about in my youth. The most famous was Louis Pasteur, the chemist who proved that microbes could cause human disease. Shortly thereafter, Robert Koch of Germany discovered the acid-fast tubercle bacillus that causes TB; Gerhard Hansen of Norway identified the acid-fast bacillus of leprosy; and Hideo Noguchi of Japan proved that spiral-shaped bacteria caused syphilis.

All these brilliant microbiologic discoveries ushered in the golden age of medicine. As a young physician, I assumed that all the bacteria which caused serious illnesses had already been discovered. Bacteria were the cause of three of man's most feared diseases: syphilis, TB and leprosy. But in medical school we were taught that cancer is not caused by bacteria.

Now that I had proved to myself that cancer microbes existed, I wanted to learn more about other scientists who had studied the cancer microbe. In my library research, I learned that "the parasite of cancer" was seriously discussed a century ago by top-notch scientists of that era.

When bacteria were discovered in TB and other infectious diseases, it was thought that bacteria might also be involved in cancer. In 1890, William Russell (1852-1940) first reported "cancer parasites" in cancer tissue that was specially stained with carbol fuchsin, a red dye. Russell, a distinguished pathologist and Professor of Clinical Medicine at Edinburgh University in Scotland, identified microbes in almost every cancer tumor he examined. The "parasite" was present inside the cells (intracellular) and outside the cells (extracellular). The smallest parasites were barely visible microscopically; and the largest parasites were as large as red blood cells. Russell also found similar parasites in tuberculosis, syphilis, and skin ulcers[6].

Other scientists were quick to refute Russell's research. In a microscopic study of cancer and TB, published in 1892, Klein concluded that Russell's parasites were not microbes but were merely large granules produced by "the assimilation of fat."[7] In 1899 Plimmer, like Russell, also discovered intra- and extracellular "parasitic bodies" in 1130 of 1278 cancer cases. He injected animals with cancer microbes and produced cancer in the animals[8]. In 1902 LeCount disputed Plimmer's so-called cancer parasites by insisting the parasites were, in reality, normal cellular structures that were "archoplasmic" in origin[9].

Russell's pleomorphic "parasites" are now called "Russell bodies" by modern day pathologists. The "bodies" are believed to be non-microbial. Researchers theorize that Russell bodies are "immunoglobulins" (protein substances) formed within the blood "plasma cells." However, in a recent electron microscopic study, Su-Ming Hsu, et al, maintain that the exact nature and origin of Russell bodies are obscure[10]. Pathologists have never considered the possibility that Russell bodies represent cell wall deficient bacteria. Further research may prove that Russell bodies are forms of the pleomorphic cancer microbe identical with Russell's "parasite of cancer."

At the close of the nineteenth century many different microbes were cultured from cancer. These microbes were variously named "cancer coccidia," "blastomycetes," "sporozoons," and "amoeboid parasites." Some of these microbes resembled Russell's parasites, and a few microbes produced cancer tumors when inoculated into animals. Because the majority of these microbes failed to produce cancer tumors in animals, most doctors considered these cancer microbes as "contaminants."

By the early part of the twentieth century the top cancer experts rejected the cancer parasite as the cause of cancer. The most influential physician to speak against the cancer microbe was James Ewing, an American pathologist and author of the widely read textbook, *NEOPLASTIC DISEASES*. In 1919 Ewing wrote that "few competent observers consider it (the parasitic theory) as a possible explanation in cancer." In Ewing's view, cancer did not act like an infection. Therefore, microbes could not possibly cause cancer. Ewing concluded, "The general facts of the genesis of tumors are strongly against the possibility of a parasitic origin."[11] His opinion was supported by other influential researchers, who were unable to produce tumors in animals by injecting them with so-called cancer parasites. As a result, the cancer parasite theory was discarded and few doctors dared to contradict Ewing's dogma by continuing the search for a cancer microbe.

James Young, an obstetrician from Scotland, refused to be intimidated. He repeatedly grew pleomorphic bacteria from breast, uterine and genital cancer, and from cancerous lymph nodes. Young readily admitted his cancer microbe was peculiar. It had a "specific life cycle" with a "spore stage" comprised of exceedingly tiny and barely visible spores. In laboratory culture these spores transformed into larger coccoid forms, yeast-like forms, and rods. Young claimed the cancer parasite was related to common bacteria which are found everywhere in nature[12].

Young's cancer microbe met with a hostile reception, particularly by Archibald Leitch, a colleague who was chosen to evaluate Young's research. Leitch claimed he couldn't confirm Young's findings of a cancer germ. A heated controversy developed, along with a hostile exchange of letters that were published in *The British Medical Journal* in 1926. In one letter Leitch proclaimed, "I do not grumble at Dr. Young's poor opinion of me, nor at his controversial methods, but I am genuinely sorry that a man of his abilities should waste his time on his so-called 'cancer parasites' — what my old teacher, Professor George Buchanan, would have described as just a wee lump of *dirt*."[13]

During the 1920s the idea of a cancer parasite was kept alive in America by John Nuzum, a Chicago physician. Nuzum consistently cultured a pleomorphic coccus from breast cancer in mice, and from human breast cancer. Some of Nuzum's cocci were tiny virus-sized forms which easily passed through a filter designed to hold back bacteria.

Nuzum could not produce experimental cancer in mice but he did succeed in producing breast cancer in two of ten female dogs that were repeatedly injected with the cocci[14]. In a dangerous human experiment he injected the groin of a 70 year-old man with cocci cultured from human breast cancer[15]. After 62 injections over an 18 week period, a skin cancer formed in the man's groin. Nuzum's human experiment showed that breast cancer microbes were also capable of producing a different kind of cancer, such as skin cancer.

In 1925 *Northwest Medicine* published two papers by Michael Scott, a Montana surgeon who learned about the cancer microbe in T.J. Glover's lab in 1921[16-17]. Scott's microbe was similar to Young's. The parasite had a life cycle composed of three stages: a coccus, a rod, and a "spore sac" stage. Scott detected the cancer microbe in cancer tissue and insisted the parasite secreted a toxin which made the body's cells cancerous.

Scott believed cancer was an infection like tuberculosis.

He wrote, "We are positive that as soon as the medical profession and laity become convinced of the infectious nature of carcinoma (cancer) and its contagiousity, the adoption of preventive mesaures, which will follow, will effect a lowering of the rate of incidence of this disease, comparable with what obtains today with tuberculosis." Scott believed an effective vaccine against cancer could be developed. He devised a promising treatment that cured some hopeless cancer patients, but his treatment methods were quickly suppressed by the medical establishment.

According to Robert Netterberg and Robert Taylor's *THE CANCER CONSPIRACY* (1981), Scott "became a forgotten man, except to those 'doomed' patients he cured of cancer. A devout Catholic, Scott tried to find research support at Catholic colleges, seeking out medical departments that would continue his experiments. But orthodoxy prevailed, the medical world ironically having become as dogmatic as the Church had been in the days of Galileo. Scott died in California in 1967, hopeful to the end"[18].

In 1929, the Stearns and B.F. Sturdivant, microbiologists in Pasadena, California, repeatedly isolated pleomorphic bacteria from cancer tumors. They could not classify the microbe because of its highly complex growth forms, which included tiny and large cocci, rods, and fungal-like forms[19].

A year later, Glover was the first to consistently isolate cancer microbes from the *blood* of cancer patients. "Old" laboratory cultures of the microbe transformed into "spore bearing bacilli" and fungi with large "spore sacs."[20]

In 1934 Wilhelm von Brehmer, a Berlin scientist, described and illustrated microbes that he observed *within the blood cells of cancer patients*[21]. Georges Mazet, a French physician, discovered pleomorphic, acid-fast bacteria in Hodgkin's disease in 1941. He later reported similar acid-fast bacteria in many different kinds of cancer, including leukemia[22-24].

In the late 1970s Guido Tedeschi, and other Italian microbiologists at the University of Camerino, discovered microbial "granules" in the red blood cells of healthy and ill people. Some of the bacteria Tedeschi cultured from the blood cells were acid-fast, a feature shared with the cancer microbe[25]. Although this research indicates bacteria exist in "normal" blood, physicians are still taught that normal blood is sterile and bacteria-free.

After learning some of the secrets of the scleroderma microbe I decided to test lupus erythematosus (LE), an "autoimmune" disease closely related to scleroderma. Tissue sections of LE were stained with Lida Mattman's acid-fast stain and acid-fast microbial forms were detected in the tissue.

In the early part of this century, physicians suspected LE might be an infection related to tuberculosis. Various bacteria such as staphylococci, streptococci, coccobacilli, and tubercle bacilli were cultured from LE tissue[26]. But like the cancer microbe work, the experts considered these microbes "contaminants" and "secondary invaders." As a result, these old microbiologic LE studies are now ignored and forgotten.

I studied the autopsy tissue of a woman who died with LE. The lupus microbe was visible in the heart, lungs, kidneys, adrenal glands, brain, and in the connective tissue[27]. Skin lesions of LE patients were cultured; and Dan Kelso and Joyce E. Jones were able to grow pleomorphic bacteria.

Joyce Jones is a microbiologist who was initially skeptical about my research. However, she offered to try to culture bacteria from scleroderma and LE skin biopsy samples in her lab. She became a believer in the work when she consistently isolated pleomorphic organisms from the diseased skin samples.

Through her daily observations of the scleroderma cultures, Joyce discovered that the scleroderma microbe defied the established rules of bacteriology. For example, orthodox microbiology teaches that cocci (such as *Staphylococcus epidermidis*) are separate and distinct from coccobacilli (such as corynebacteria); and no relationship is supposed to exist between these two different microbes. But Joyce discovered that the pure *Staphylococcus epidermidis* (coccus) form of the scleroderma microbe transformed into corynebacteria (rods and cocci). This transformation was dependent on the laboratory medium Joyce used to feed the microbe. Conversely, when Joyce changed the growth medium the corynebacterial microbes (rods and cocci) transformed back to pure staphylococci (cocci only).

According to traditional microbiological dogma, all this changing back and forth between two "different" microbes is an impossibility. According to the "rules," this is not supposed to happen! Nevertheless, Joyce proved that the precise identification and classification of the scleroderma microbe depended on what it was fed in the laboratory.

For several years Dan, Joyce, and I carefully studied a scleroderma microbe that we repeatedly cultured from a young Asian-American woman with a debilitating form of scleroderma called "pansclerotic morphea." Not only did the microbe vacillate back and forth between a staphylococcal and a corynebacterial organism, it also became fungus-like! In the scleroderma tissue sections we detected many coccus forms of the microbe and a few rod-shaped bacteria. In 1984 the *Archives of Dermatology* published the bacteriologic findings in this case, including eleven photos of the cultured pleomorphic scleroderma microbe, and four photos of the microbe in the tissue sections[28]. *The International Journal of Dermatology* also published two papers of our scleroderma and lupus research, along with numerous photos of the microbes we discovered in these diseases[26, 29].

After twenty years of hunting microbes in skin diseases, I knew the old established "rules" of microbiology were not workable. Bacteriologists loved to classify microbes into neat little boxes so that they could study them more effectively. But the classification system had nothing to do with the way microbes acted "in nature." In nature, bacteria constantly change form. Pleomorphic scleroderma and cancer microbes are impossible to classify because they defy the dogma of microbiology. In reality, the bacteriologists' classification system makes it utterly impossible to understand the cancer microbe.

Nevertheless, the microbiology experts insist that microbes be carefully classified and categorized. Not surprisingly, microbiologists have litle interest in pleomorphic microbes that are not "stable." By definition, pleomorphic organisms are unstable microbes. Consequently, pleomorphic microbes are often dismissed as "contaminants" unworthy of further investigation.

In my experience, pleomorphic TB and scleroderma and cancer microbes resemble ordinary microbes such as staphylococci, corynebacteria (diphtheroids), yeast-like microbes, or fungi. In tissue, the granular and coccoid-shaped microbes are found inside the cells (intracellular) and outside the cells (extracellular). The microbes can transform into larger structures that microbiologists and pathologists have named "large bodies" or "Russell bodies" or "hematoxylin bodies." Without a knowledge of the actual growth potential of cell wall deficient pleomorphic forms, it is difficult for doctors to accept these "large bodies" as microbes.

Of course, all this is heresy to orthodox microbiologists, virologists, pathologists, oncologists, hematologists, infectious disease specialists and dermatologists. It is sad that these specialists do not have the necessary laboratory experience and the open-mindedness to appreciate the findings of researchers who have studied pleomorphic organisms and the microbiology of cancer. Historically, it has been easier to label these scientists as "quacks."

I had hoped that my cancer research would stimulate other physicians and microbiologists to prove or disprove my findings but, as usual, the work was generally ignored. The idea of bacteria as the cause of cancer and "autoimmune" diseases is considered too preposterous. Dermatologists have been carefully taught that scleroderma and LE are diseases "of unknown etiology." And the cancer experts are secure and comfortable in their certainty that cancer is not caused by bacteria.

While the biomedical world eagerly awaits the discovery of an etiologic agent in cancer, and while cancer scientists plead for more money for research, a century of cancer microbe research remains ignored. It is ironic to learn that the real dogma of orthodox medical science is: SEEK BUT DO NOT FIND!

In my research I had discovered too much. Initially, the research committee was willing to grant funds for my scleroderma studies. Scleroderma is an obscure disease that few doctors care about. However, when I began to study cancer and AIDS, the committee balked. Through the hospital grapevine, I heard I was encroaching too heavily on the territory of the bacteriologists and pathologists. It was considered audacious and unorthodox for a dermatologist to study cancer, especially autopsied cases.

In desperation, the committee insisted on a statistical analysis of my research and demanded that I meet with their statistician. I was dumbfounded. What did statistics have to do with cancer microbe research? The statistician assured me he could devise and authorize an autopsy research project that would meet the committee's requirements. The committee obviously wanted to control my research, and I could not argue with their decision.

A statistical project of autopsied tissue was set up which was doomed from the start. The project required cooperation and expertise from the pathology department. But unfortunately, none of the pathologists had any knowledge of the cancer microbe, nor did they recognize it in diseased tissue. I myself was at a loss to evaluate the study because I had seen the microbe in "normal" tissue, a point which left the statistician baffled. Physicians believe that disease germs should be found only in diseased tissue, but never in "normal" tissue.

I had to face the fact that my cancer microbe work was incomprehensible to my colleagues. Doctors are taught that each infectious disease is caused by a specific microbe. But the scleroderma microbe and the lupus microbe and the sarcoidosis microbe and the cancer microbe all looked and acted the same. The doctors said it was impossible for the same appearing germ to be involved in so many different cancerous and non-cancerous diseases. My cancer microbe research didn't make any sense.

I knew there were inconsistencies and improbabilities in my research, but I firmly believed the cancer microbe was involved in cancer. It was true that I had occasionally seen small numbers of the microbe in "normal" tissue. But when tissue became "precancerous," the microbes increased in number. And when patients died from cancer, their tissues were overrun with cancer microbes. I studied autopsies of cancer patients who had been treated with massive doses of antibiotics for weeks before death: the antibiotics failed to kill the cancer microbes. I saw the microbe in tissue that had been burned with massive doses of radiation therapy. I saw the microbe thriving in cancerous tissue that had been blitzed with chemotherapy; the cancer cells were destroyed, but the cancer microbe remained! Nothing fazed the cancer microbe: not surgery, not radiation, not antibiotics, not chemotherapy. The cancer microbe was indestructible!

In the early 1970s, Virginia discovered that the cancer microbe secretes a hormone called human choriogonadotropic hormone (HCG)[30]. The hormone protects the cancer microbe from destruction by the immune system and allows the microbe to incite the cancer process. Virginia also claims the cancer microbe (*Progenitor cryptocides*) is present inside sperm cells. At the moment of conception (when the sperm cell impregnates the egg), the cancer microbe inside the sperm cell releases the HCG hormone. The HGC hormone protects the fertilized egg. This hormone protection is vital because half the genetic material in the fertilized egg is "foreign" genetic material supplied by the father's genes in the sperm cell.

Without HCG hormone protection, the mother's immune cells would destroy the embryo containing the father's foreign genetic material. The continual secretion of HCG hormone allows the fetus to survive. Through this reproductive function, Virginia believes the cancer microbe allows life to recreate itself constantly.

Virginia also claims the cancer microbe lives in every cell. When cells are damaged, the hormone-secreting cancer microbe aids in healing. Under unhealthy conditions the microbe induces cancer and other diseases. The microbiology of cancer is difficult to explain because the "facts" of the cancer microbe seriously conflict with the rigid orthodox teachings of modern day microbiology.

When Pasteur popularized germs a century ago, the science of medicine entered a new era. After many centuries of ignorance, physicians finally accepted the idea that microscopic germs could cause human disease. Tragically, the principles of infectious disease that were popularized during Pasteur's time have made doctors blind to the most important microbe of all — the cancer microbe.

A few years ago I learned of a French physician who tried to teach nineteenth-century doctors about other "forces" that were operative in infectious and cancerous diseases. When I studied the achievements of this forgotten scientist, I discovered there was much more to cancer than the cancer microbe.

The cancer microbe was only a key that unlocked a realm of long-suppressed scientific discoveries that delved into the origin of life itself.

A realm in which life and death exist simultaneously!

References:

1. **Cantwell AR Jr, Kelso DW**: Microbial findings in cancer of the breast and in their metastases to the skin. J Dermatol Surg Oncol 7: 483-491, 1981.

2. **Cantwell AR Jr**: Variably acid-fast bacteria in a rare case of coexistent malignant lymphoma and cutaneous sarcoid-like granulomas. Intl J Dermatol 21: 99-106, 1982.

3. **Cantwell AR Jr**: Histologic observations of variably acid-fast coccoid forms suggestive of cell wall deficient bacteria in Hodgkin's disease. A report of four cases. Growth 45: 168- 187, 1981.

4. **Cantwell AR Jr**: Variably acid-fast pleomorphic bacteria as a possible cause of mycosis fungoides. J Dermatol Surg Oncol 8: 203-213, 1982.

5. **Cantwell AR Jr, Lawson JW**: Necroscopic findings of pleomorphic, variably acid-fast bacteria in a fatal case of Kaposi's sarcoma. J Dermatol Surg Oncol 7: 923-930, 1981.

6. **Russell W**: An address on a characteristic organism of cancer. Brit Med J 2: 1356-1360, 1890.

7. **Klein R**: Ueber die Beziehung der Russell'schen Fuchsinkorperchen zu den Altman'schen Zellgranulis. Ziegler's Beitrage Z Patho Anat 11: 125-144, 1892.

8. **Plimmer HG**: On the aetiology and histology of cancer, with special reference to recent work on the subject. Practitioner 62: 430-455, 1899.

9. **LeCount ER**: The analogies between Plimmer's bodies and certain structures found normally in the cytoplasm. J Med Res 7: 383-393, 1902.

10. **Hsu SM, Hsu PL, McMillan PN, et al**: Russell bodies. A light and electron microscopic immunoperoxidase study. Amer J Clin Path 77: 26-31, 1982.

11. **Ewing J**: The parasitic theory. In, Ewing J (Ed): *Neoplastic Diseases*, Ed 1. Philadelphia, Saunders, 1919, pp 114-126.

12. **Young J**: Description of an organism obtained from carcinomatous growths. Edinburgh Med J (New Series) 27: 212- 221, 1921.

13. **Leitch A**: Dr. Young's cancer parasite. Brit Med J, April 17, 1926, p 721.

14. **Nuzum JW**: A critical study of an organism associated with a transplantable carcinoma of the white mouse. Surg Gynecol Obstet 33: 167-175. 1921.

15. **Nuzum JW**: The experimental production of metastasizing carcinoma of the breast of the dog and primary epithelioma in man by repeated inoculation of a micrococcus isolated from human breast cancer. Surg Gynecol Obstet 11: 343-352, 1925.

16. **Scott MJ**: The parasitic origin of carcinoma. Northwest Med 24: 162-166, 1925.

17. **Scott MJ**: More about the parasitic origin of malignant epithelial growths. Northwest Med 25: 492-498, 1925.

18. **Netterberg RE, Taylor RT**: *The Cancer Conspiracy.* Pinnacle Books, New York, 1981.

19. **Stearn EW, Sturdivant BF, Stearn AE**: The ontogeny of an organism isolated from malignant tumors. J Bacteriol 18: 227- 245, 1929.

20. **Glover TJ**: The bacteriology of cancer. Canada Lancet Pract 75: 92-111, 1930.

21. **Von Brehmer W**: "Siphonospora poymorphia" n. sp., neuer Mikroorganismus des Blutes und seine Beziehung zur Tumorigenese. Med Welt 8: 1179-1185, 1934.

22. **Mazet G**: Etude bacteriologiques sur la malade d'Hodgkin. Montpellier Med 1941: 316-328, 1941.

23. **Mazet G**: Presence d'elements alcoolo-acido-resistants dans les moelles leucemiques et les moelles non leucemiques. Semaine des Hopitaux, No. 1, 2, 1962, pp 35-38.

24. **Mazet G**: Corynebacterium, tubercle bacillus and cancer. Growth 38: 61-74, 1974.

25. **Tedeschi GG, Bondi A, Paparelli M, et al**: Electron microscopical evidence of the evolution of coryne-bacteria- like microbes within human erythrocytes. Experientia 34: 458- 460, 1978.

26. **Cantwell AR Jr, Kelso DW, Jones JE**: Histologic observations of coccoid forms suggestive of cell wall deficient bacteria in cutaneous and systemic lupus erythematosus. Intl J Dermatol 21: 526-537, 1982.

27. **Cantwell AR Jr, Cove JK**: Variably acid-fast bacteria in a necropsied case of systemic lupus

erythematosus with acute myocardial infarction. Cutis 33: 560-567, 1984.

28. **Cantwell AR Jr**: Histologic observations of pleomorphic, variably acid-fast bacteria in scleroderma, morphea, and lichen sclerosus et atrophicus. Intl J Dermatol 23: 45-52, 1984.

29. **Cantwell AR Jr, Jones JE, Kelso DW**: Pleomorphic, variably acid-fast bacteria in an adult patient with disabling pansclerotic morphea. Arch Dermatol 120: 656-661, 1983.

30. **Livingston VWC, Livingston AM**: Some cultural, immunological, and biochemical properties of *Progenitor cryptocides*. Trans NY Acad Sci 36, Series 2, No. 6, 1974, pp 569-582. 1974.

CHAPTER NINE

Bechamp's Microzymas

As I found myself more and more alienated from my peers in medicine, I became intrigued by some of the adventurous people and scientists I encountered in the field of so-called alternative, holistic and unorthodox medicine. They were an odd mix of people and only a few were MDs. However, they were brought together by the belief that healing was best obtained by combining the forces of mind, body, and spirit. I had no trouble dealing with this concept because it was exactly what Edgar Cayce talked about in his psychic readings back in the 1930s.

My formal initiation into unorthodox medicine took place in the summer of 1985 when Lorraine Rosenthal of the Cancer Control Society (CCS) invited me to speak about my AIDS research at its annual convention in Los Angeles. Virginia Livingston was also scheduled to appear on the program. The CCS is a controversial educational organization that brings information on alternative cancer treatment to the attention of the public. Many of these treatment methods have been condemned by the medical establishment.

I knew it could be the "kiss of death" to speak at the CCS meeting. I had already gotten in trouble for lecturing at a medical symposium sponsored by Virginia Livingston's San Diego Clinic. A physician in my medical group became angry when he noticed my name and affiliation in a *Los Angeles Times* newspaper advertisement for the meeting. The doctor complained to the hospital administrators who demanded to know why I was associating with a known "quack" like Virginia Livingston. They were angry that I did not seek their approval to speak at her symposium. I explained I had lectured on my research to health professionals for over twenty years; I never asked for "approval" because I didn't know it was required. Despite my objections I was emphatically told that, in the future, I could never publicly declare my affiliation with the Medical Group unless permission was officially granted.

I lectured at the CCS, carefully concealing my medical affiliation from the program. I was eager to speak about cancer bacteria in AIDS. I had previously lectured on the subject but my AIDS research evoked little interest because the top experts were interested in viruses in AIDS — not bacteria.

Lorraine warned me that the AMA always had reporters covering the convention. I could care less; I hated being intimidated. During my lecture I showed slides of cancer microbes that were discovered in the diseased and cancerous tissue of gay men with AIDS. I also showed the bacteria that were cultured from the Kaposi's sarcoma skin tumors, and from the blood of AIDS patients. Slides of the cancer microbe in breast cancer, skin cancer, lymphoma, and other types of cancer were also presented. Virginia Livingston talked about her thirty-eight year experience with the cancer microbe, and how the patient's immune system could be strengthened to fight the microbe.

None of the local news media mentioned our presentations, but the AMA-sponsored *American Medical News* (August 9, 1985) reported on the convention. Helene

Brown, a spokesperson for the American Cancer Society, branded the CCS as "a new dimension in murder." She claimed that quack cures denied cancer patients life-saving treatments. The AMA reporter, Lisa Krieger, put down my presentation of cancer microbes as a show of "purple blotches." She wrote: "These cancer microbes can be seen in AIDS patients, claimed Alan Cantwell MD, a dermatologist in group practice in Los Angeles. He said he had isolated 'intracellular parasites' from the heart, lung, and intestines of AIDS patients. 'It looks like a germ, grows like a germ, and kills like a germ,' he said, pointing to purple blotches on a photo of a microscopic slide."

Krieger's report was inaccurate and misleading. I never claimed to "isolate" germs from AIDS autopsy tissue. However, I did show cancer microbes in the autopsy tissue specimens. Two years earlier, photographs of these post-mortem findings of AIDS bacteria were published in the scientific journal *Growth*[1].

At the CCS physician's symposium, I met Roy Kupsinel MD from Olviedo, Florida. Roy was certain my cancer microbe work was related to the work of a scientist named Bechamp, but I explained that I had never heard of his research. Roy explained there was a book about Bechamp. He promised to send me details on where I could purchase it.

Within a few days, Roy's letter arrived. The name of the book was *BECHAMP OR PASTEUR?* by E. Douglas Hume. It was available from a small publisher in Milwaukee, but Roy didn't have the address. I put the letter aside, and forgot about Bechamp.

Weeks later I was delivering copies of my book, *AIDS: THE MYSTERY AND THE SOLUTION*, to the CCS headquarters in Hollywood. Lorraine Rosenthal manages the book department which supplies members with alternative health books. As I placed my books on her desk, she said, "I just received six copies of a reprinted book on Bechamp from the Lee Foundation in Milwaukee. He is an interesting scientist. You should buy a copy. It's only $19.00 and it's a hard book to find."

Now that Bechamp's book had found me, I couldn't refuse Lorraine's offer. Besides, I was curious to find out how Bechamp's research could possibly be related to mine.

When I first read *BECHAMP OR PASTEUR?* it was rather dull and uninspiring. Only with several forced rereadings did I slowly discover that Bechamp's strange ideas were compelling me to reassess my own dogmatic beliefs about the origin and nature of the cancer microbe.

BECHAMP OR PASTEUR? A LOST CHAPTER IN THE HISTORY OF BIOLOGY[2] was first published in England in 1923. Ethel Douglas Hume wrote the book at the request of Montague Leverson, a Baltimore physician who was deeply attracted to Bechamp's ideas. Leverson considered Bechamp a scientific genius whose discoveries could revolutionize medicine.

Bechamp (1816-1908) had an incredible list of scientific appointments at French universities: Doctor of Science, Doctor of Medicine, Professor of Medical Chemistry and Pharmacy at Montpelier, Professor of Physics and Toxicology at Strasbourg, Professor of Biological Chemistry and Dean of Medicine at Lille, Professor of Physics, Professor of Toxicology, Professor of Medical Chemistry and Pharmacy, and Professor of Biological Chemistry. When he died, the *Moniteur*

Scientifique devoted eight pages to listing Bechamp's writings and credentials. After his death, his work slowly disappeared from the science books and journals. In time, the eradication of Bechamp was complete.

During his lifetime Bechamp was overshadowed by Louis Pasteur (1822-1895), the most celebrated scientist of the nineteenth century. Both men were highly-regarded members of the French Academy of Science, and each submitted their scientific findings to the Academy for review and publication. Unfortunately, the ideas of Bechamp and Pasteur clashed with a vengeance. The intense professional rivalry between the two scientists is recorded in the proceedings of the *Comptes Rendus*, the official journal of the Academy.

According to Hume, the records of the *Comptes Rendus* prove that many of Pasteur's brilliant discoveries were actually previous discoveries of Bechamp. Apparently, Pasteur had a nasty habit of stealing the work of other scientists. After cleverly disguising it, he subsequently declared the work as his own. Hume writes that many of Bechamp's experiments clearly take precedence over Pasteur's, even though Pasteur was given the credit. Because Bechamp frequently criticized Pasteur's scientific work, the feud between the two men intensified in the Academy.

Despite the controversy, the Academy basked in the glow of Pasteur's worldwide fame. No matter how carefully Bechamp argued against Pasteur's scientific methods and conclusions, the Academy always gave the nod to their favorite son. There was no way Bechamp's ideas could win against the powerful Pasteur.

Born six years after Bechamp, Pasteur was destined for greatness. As a chemist, he lacked Bechamp's amazing professional accreditations in the fields of biology, physics, and pharmacology. Most importantly, Pasteur had no medical training and lacked Bechamp's understanding of disease pathology. Nevertheless, Pasteur had the necessary ingredients for worldly success. Born under the intensely ambitious sign of Capricorn, he was determined to be the world's most famous scientist. And through his discoveries, he established the essential political connections that extended as high up as the Emperor of France.

Pasteur allowed no one to stand in his way, and certainly not Bechamp. In his ascent to scientific stardom, he plagiarized Bechamp's experiments and ideas, and twisted them to suit his own scientific and political agenda. Through the mastery of power politics, Pasteur rose to the highest position in academia. . . and Bechamp's important experiments and theories were forgotten. Ultimately, the chemist became known as the "Father of modern medicine."

The times favored Pasteur because his ideas were in tune with the science and the politics of his day. . . and Bechamp's were not. The light of history shone brilliantly on Pasteur, and eclipsed Bechamp completely.

The nineteenth century scientific world of Pasteur and Bechamp was a time when doctors practiced medicine without knowledge of infectious microbes. Microbes were discovered a century and a half earlier, but only a few scientists suspected these strange-looking "animalcules" could cause human disease. Physicians scoffed at such foolishness. How could tiny microscopic creatures cause a grown man to become sick? The idea was laughable!

Nineteenth century scientists focused their energy on questions like: Where did life come from? What caused death and decay? What caused the transformation of sugar cane into alcohol? Why did wine turn to vinegar? What was the mysterious nature of fermentation? What caused organic material to decay and putrify? Why did milk turn sour? Why did meat spoil?

Scientists who worked with lenses knew that hay placed in water gave rise to new life. Within two weeks this hay-water infusion gave birth to animalcules. There was a suspected "force" in the hay-water mixture that produced new life by a process known as "spontaneous regeneration."

At age twenty-six, Pasteur began his brilliant career in chemistry by discovering four different molecular structures of tartaric acid, instead of two as was previously thought. He cleverly realized the commercial value of his biochemical research. Consequently, when beet-farmers asked him to investigate the mysteries of sugar beet production, Pasteur responded enthusiastically. In the process of fermentation, beets turn into sugar and alcohol. The beet farmers' problem was simple: How could the commercial yield of alcohol be increased? Before long, Pasteur was peering energetically into microscopes in order to study the microbes (animalcules) in the brew of the beet infusions.

As his knowledge of fermentation and microbes increased, Pasteur's conclusions ran afoul of other scientists who believed that microbes arose "spontaneously" in fermentations. Pasteur discovered that microbes did not appear spontaneously in infusions if air and air-dust particles were totally removed, nor did fermentation take place.

Pasteur concluded that fermentation was caused by air germs. When air germs were excluded, fermentation and putrifaction could not take place. The chemist assured the beet farmers that they could make more money if they modified the beet fermentation process in ways that would control the germs in the air.

Pasteur was a master of self-promotion, greatly popularizing his research by stressing the importance of microbes in the agricultural industry. His successful experiments undertaken for the silkworm and the beer industry made Pasteur a national hero.

The idea that microbes cause disease did not originate with Pasteur, but he was determined to show that air germs were the cause of human disease. To prove this, Pasteur devised a series of experiments to disprove the popular theory of spontaneous generation. In Pasteur's view, the germs of death and decay came only from the air; never from a "force" within the cells.

Pasteur presented his experimental data to the Academy for approval. The members concurred; and the theory of spontaneous generation was overthrown. Soon Pasteur proclaimed, "Life is a germ, and a germ is life." Later, he added: "A disease is a germ and a germ is a disease." Pasteur made it all quite simple.

Only a few scientists objected to Pasteur's new dogma. Bechamp agreed that air microbes were important in fermentations. However, as a physician, microbiologist, chemist, physicist, microscopist, and as a cellular cytologist, Bechamp had studied various human, animal and plant diseases. Pasteur was ignoring other vitally important factors that were involved in fermentation and disease.

Henry Charleton Bastian, an English biologist and microscopist, also disagreed vehemently with Pasteur. Bastian had authored two successful books: *THE EVOLUTION OF LIFE* (1872), and *EVOLUTION AND THE ORIGIN OF LIFE* (1874). The biologist frequently observed microbes change form, transforming from one species into another. He saw microbes develop deep within the core of fruits and vegetables, and even within the bowels of ancient rock and limestone. These microbes could never have originated from air germs because it was impossible for air germs to penetrate these substances from the outside. Pasteur may have convinced the Academy, but he certainly didn't fool scientists like Bechamp, Bastian, and others. There were holes in Pasteur's experiments that could not be covered up, no matter how impressive his showmanship. According to the outspoken Professor Bastian, the mighty Pasteur did not succeed in striking a "mortal blow" to the theory of spontanous regeneration.

The *Comptes Rendus* records indicate that Bechamp was always a step ahead of Pasteur, even though Pasteur was always given the credit and the limelight. Pasteur clarified the mystery of fermentation by demonstrating air germs, but Bechamp's experiments had showed the same thing two years earlier. And Bechamp first proved that air germs could not ferment an infusion of cane sugar if creosote was added to the infusion. Bechamp was also the first to correctly diagnose the true nature of silkworm disease; and eight years before Pasteur, Bechamp proved that germs growing on the surface of grapes were the microbes involved in wine fermentation.

During his many years of experimentation, Bechamp made his most brilliant discovery: THE DISCOVERY OF MICROZYMAS! There was nothing Pasteur hated more than the cursed microzyma theory that Bechamp was proclaiming. With Bechamp as his most outspoken scientific rival in the Academy, Pasteur would have to make sure that Bechamp and his damned microzymas were obliterated from the annals of science.

To a large extent, Pasteur succeeded in destroying

Bechamp and his work. But Bechamp's destruction was
not complete. Fate offered Bechamp one last hope for
scientific immortality — in the guise of Montague
Leverson, an American physician from Baltimore,
Maryland.

———

In 1908 Bechamp was eighty-six years old, and Leverson
was over seventy. Time was running out for both men.
Two weeks before Bechamp's death, Leverson met him
in Paris. During their brief time together, Bechamp
dictated his life's work to Leverson. The meeting was
fortunate and fruitful for the history of medicine.

After Bechamp's death, Leverson translated Bechamp's
writings into English. In 1912, Antoine Bechamp's *THE
BLOOD AND ITS THIRD ANATOMICAL ELE-
MENT* was published in London[3]. Through Ethel
Douglas Hume's association with Dr. Leverson, her
book *BECHAMP OR PASTEUR?* was published a
decade later in London. Both books comprise the
"essential" Bechamp.

The beginning chapters of Hume's book detail the
nineteenth century fermentation experiments of Bechamp
and Pasteur. Pasteur's fermentation studies had a
profound effect on biomedical thought by laying the
scientific foundation for twentieth century medicine,
biochemistry and microbiology.

Hume repeatedly insists the records prove that
Bechamp, not Pasteur, was the first to discover (in 1857)
that air-borne organisms cause fermentation. Yet Pasteur
was credited for the discovery! Although this was
interesting, I wondered what all this had to do with
cancer microbe research. A third of the way through the

book, Hume explains Bechamp's discovery of microzymas; and I slowly became aware that this discovery was the "connection" to my cancer microbe research.

In the 1860s, Bechamp claimed that the microzyma is the essential unit of life. It is this microzymian theory that put Bechamp into direct conflict with Pasteur and his allies in the Academy.

Bechamp excelled as a microscopist and cytologist (a specialist in the study of cells). Inside the cells he observed the tiny, round, granular bodies which glistened as tiny sparkles of refracted light. He was not the first to see the granules, but he was the first to suspect that these "little bodies" might hold the key to the origin of life. Other scientists who studied the "little bodies" named them "scintillating corpuscles" and "molecular granulations." Later, they were called "microsomes" and "chromatin granules." Bechamp passionately explored the nature and function of these glistening granules that were contained within all living cells.

Bechamp studied microzymas in various diseases, including tuberculosis. In TB, the unhealthy cells contained large numbers of granules. His varied academic background in medicine, chemistry, and physics, and his special expertise in the use of polarized light, allowed Bechamp to devise a series of unique biological experiments to study microzymas. Bechamp's experiments showed that *microzymas are tiny chemical factories which have the ability to ferment.*

He named microzymas after Greek words meaning "small" and "ferment." Bechamp's chemical tests proved microzymas were insoluble in water. Composed of hydrogen, carbon, and other elements, the microzymas produced nucleic acid. When Bechamp heated the little bodies to high temperatures they lost their ability to ferment.

The microzymas were alive and teemed with chemically active energy. Bechamp declared that microzymas were essential and indispensible anatomic cellular elements which digested, transformed, and assimilated nutrients required by the cells. Bechamp tried to kill microzymas, but they proved indestructible. He studied them in all sorts of tissue and organic matter, in chalk, plant life, and in yeasts. They were present in the amoeba, the smallest form of animal life; and in the bacteria, the smallest form of plant life. He studied the microzymas in healthy and diseased human cells. Bechamp learned that microzymas of each organ behave differently from one another. For example, the little granular bodies of the liver had different biochemical properties than those of the kidney. In addition, microzymas in the organs of young people differed biochemically from microzymas in old people.

Bechamp made a tremendous scientific discovery. Under certain conditions (and by a process called "vibrionen evolution") Bechamp watched microzymas transform into bacteria! First, the microzymas enlarged into round coccoid forms. Then the round forms might couple into two or more units; or they might sprout into rods. Bechamp was positive the "little bodies" were involved in the fermentation process, and in the production of disease!

Where do microzymas come from? Bechamp startled the scientific world by declaring, "They are the organized and yet living remains of beings that lived in long past ages. They are the transmitters of heredity. Within the chromatin material of the human sperm cell are contained all the microzymian granules needed to genetically reproduce all the different cells essential for the reproduction of the human species."

Bechamp's declaration was a direct affront to Pasteur's dogma that all disease was due to air germs. Bechamp challenged the chemist by reiterating the aphorism of Pidoux: "Disease is born of us and in us." Bechamp taught that in disease the microzymas change. When deprived of proper nutrition, microzymas might transform into bacteria by the process of "vibrionen evolution." Although normal and diseased microzymas can look the same microscopically, their biochemical functions are different.

According to Bechamp, the air germs come from microzymas (or their transformed microbial forms) that originate in diseased cells. Pasteur's so-called "air disease germs" are merely the remains of decaying matter which are picked up by the wind and scattered within the dust particles of the atmosphere.

In the hallowed walls of the French Academy, Bechamp insisted Pasteur's teaching was wrong! Bechamp declared: MICROBES ARE THE RESULT OF DISEASE, NOT THE CAUSE!!

Pasteur had supposedly proved that all disease was "exogenous" in nature. He preached that disease came from germs originating outside the body — from exposure of the body to the disease-producing air-germs. The exogenous air germs were the "only" source of fermentation and disease. According to the chemist, the body was merely a chemical complex. In Pasteur's view, a healthy body is invulnerable to foreign germs. And he taught that a healthy body contains no lethal germs!

The microzyma theory was heresy! And Bechamp's voice was drowned out by the thunderous applause for Pasteur. The doctors believed the chemist, and ignored

Bechamp. To this day, the followers of Pasteur teach medical students and microbiologists that bacteria do not change form. A coccus is a coccus is a coccus. A rod is a rod is a rod. The form of bacteria is inviolate.

The scientists of Pasteur's time also believed that the essential unit of life was the cell; and the cell was considered the smallest unit of life. Therefore, there could be no such thing as microzymas. But Bechamp knew better. He studied the cells *after* they died, and he watched the microzymas arise from the dying cells. He saw the microzymas come together to form new cells. The cells were destructible; but the microzymas were indestructible!

It took many months for me to appreciate fully the profound significance of Hume's book. Pasteur's errone-ous "germ theory of disease" became the dogma that gave birth to twentieth century "modern" medical science. Medical students are taught to venerate the correctness of Pasteurian thought, and only a fool would dare disagree with the chemist's belief that only air germs produce disease. The logic of Pasteur was very simple. And according to Bechamp, very wrong.

During the 1870s Pasteur's microbe discoveries stimu-lated the interest of Robert Koch, a young German country doctor. Like Pasteur and Bechamp, Koch had a keen interest in microbe hunting. He learned to grow microbes on potato skins, and subsequently devised special nutrients upon which disease germs could be cultured. In 1882 Koch discovered the tubercle bacillus, the microbe of tuberculosis (TB).

Robert Koch became the leading scientist of Germany. He grew TB microbes from sick patients and injected the bacteria into animals. The animals became sick and

died, and Koch recultured the TB microbes from the
diseased tissue of the animals. Koch's animal experiments proved that TB germs cause TB. Since that time,
Koch's "postulates" have become the tried-and-true
animal experimental method for proving the germ theory
of disease. However, in certain infectious diseases such
as syphilis, leprosy and AIDS, Koch's postulates have
never been proven.

Over the next century, billions of laboratory animals
were tortured and sacrificed in experiments proving and
reproving Pasteur and Koch's contention that air germs
were at the root of all human disease. With Koch's
discoveries added to Pasteur's, the "germ theory of
disease" was set in stone. The medical profession was
totally won over by the science of these two men; the
science of microbiology was born, and the study of
infectious disease commenced.

A name was needed for Pasteur's air germs. The word
"microbe" became popular. What was the "origin" of
these microbes? The answer was simple: microbes
originated eons ago when all life in the world was
formed! The Church was especially pleased with this
answer because scientists finally confirmed what had
been written in the Bible two thousand years ago.

Bechamp complained that Pasteur and Koch taught
that air germs caused disease, but their experiments
never proved it. None of their laboratory animals got TB
by breathing in air germs. They were killed by germs
Koch grew artificially in the laboratory. Koch's deadly
TB germs were always obtained from diseased tissue in
which the microzymas were already transformed into
bacteria. The disease-altered microzymas gave rise to the
disease, not the bacteria. Why couldn't doctors recognize
microzymas and understand that? Why couldn't they

comprehend that microzymas are the indestructible anatomic basis of all life?

Years before, Bechamp had killed a kitten and laid its body on a bed of carbonated lime that was mixed with creosote to prevent fermentation and putrefaction. On top of the kitten's body he added another thick layer of lime and creosote. He carefully placed all this material in a specially-made glass jar. Bechamp covered the top of the jar with layers of paper which allowed the air to seep in, but which kept out the air dust particles containing the air germs. For six years Bechamp observed the specimen. To be doubly sure of his observations and results, he repeated the experiment a second time.

At the end of the long experiment Bechamp examined the kitten's remains. The cells of the cat's organs had disappeared. In their place were the glistening granules of the indestructible microzymas. In some areas the microzymas had transformed themselves into bacteria. It was impossible for these bacteria to have originated from air-dust germs. Thereafter, Bechamp taught that all life arises from microzymas. From the dust of death, new life always arises. Bechamp's profound concept did not impress the scientists of his day, or the Church.

Bechamp believed that every microbe originated from microzymas in living cells. If diseases always came from breathing in air microbes, as Pasteur claimed, none of us would be alive. We would all be at the mercy of the many different species of deadly germs that forever lived and multiplied in the air. In times of epidemic, none of us would be spared.

Pasteur was the genius of his day; and Bechamp's microzymian theory and contrary views were an annoyance to the Academy. The establishment knew how to deal with rebels like Bechamp. His work would be ignored by the "authorities" and never cited by the "experts." His ideas would never be taken seriously in journals and textbooks. Biomedical editors would purge his name from the pages of their scientific publications. Bechamp would quickly vanish from the annals of science. This is the way all medical rebels are silenced by the establishment.

A century later, a handful of people keep Bechamp's work alive. After reading Hume's book, I wanted to know if the "little bodies" were related to scleroderma, cancer and AIDS microbes I had studied. Were any nineteenth-century photographs or drawings available that showed the appearance of microzymas?

I wrote Roy Kupsinel, but my questions were beyond his ken. He suggested I contact Glen Dettman, a microbiologist who supervised a pathology laboratory in Victoria, Australia. I sent Dettman my AIDS book and my scientific papers, along with questions about Bechamp.

A letter from "down under" arrived in May 1986. Glen was familiar with Virginia Livingston's research, but he interpreted her cancer microbe (*Progenitor cryptocides*) as a "rediscovery" of Bechamp's microzymas. He urged me to read Bechamp's THE BLOOD, available from the U.S. Library of Congress. "In THE BLOOD you will find that Bechamp referred to his 'little bodies' arranging themselves in the form of a figure eight. He also describes with great accuracy the mode of enzymes and even gives a vivid description of his genetic engineering, carried out upon yeasts. Truly an incredible genius, far ahead of his time. It is easily explainable how Pasteur's germ theory was accepted because Bechamp's peers (and tricky Louis P.) didn't have the slightest understanding of Bechamp's important research findings."

Glen and his son Ian had repeatedly seen microzymas and *Progenitor cryptocides* in dark-field microscopic examinations of the blood. Were the little bodies related to cancer microbes? Glen responded: "You ask me if what you are seeing are microzymas and I would say *yes*. However, to convince your colleagues of this is an unenviable task."

In closing, Glen hoped I would follow through on my investigation of Bechamp. "I do not have to warn you that you will receive plenty of flack, but what's flack when you have an atomic bomb to release? I wish you ultimate success."

I ordered *THE BLOOD* from the medical library, explaining that it was a rare old book available from the Library of Congress. I heard nothing for weeks. Finally, the librarian informed me the book was "unavailable" and could not be obtained anywhere. If Washington didn't have a copy, that was the end of the line.

I wrote Glen to stop referencing people to the Library of Congress. Bechamp's *BLOOD* was no longer there. The eclipse of Bechamp was complete in America.

References:

1. **Cantwell AR Jr**: Necroscopic findings of variably acid-fast bacteria in a fatal case of acquired immunodeficiency syndrome. Growth 47: 129-134, 1983.

2. **Hume ED**: *Bechamp or Pasteur?: A Lost Chapter in the History of Biology.* CW Daniel Co. Ltd., Ashington, England, 1923. (Available from The Lee Foundation for Nutritional Research, 2023 West Wisconsin Avenue, Milwaukee, Wisconsin 53201).

CHAPTER TEN

Bechamp or Pasteur?

Glen Dettman suggested I contact Dorothy Knafelc for additional information on Antoine Bechamp. He wrote, "Dorothy is a scholarly woman and a good friend who is exceedingly well-informed about Bechamp. She has made a greater study of Bechamp than any other person I know. More importantly she understands his work and is able to impart her information to others. If you care to write her about almost any aspect of Bechamp's research, you will be suitably rewarded."

In August 1986 I wrote Dorothy Knafelc in Queensland, Australia, and she responded with a beautifully hand-written letter. "I would like to explain that I am not a scientist, laboratory technician, nor do I hold any university degrees. However, I have always taken a keen interest in the subjects of biology, physics, and medicine. Self-educating by prodigious reading of scientific books, and all sorts of publications. Over thirty years ago, whilst we were living in London, my favorite British Museum Library offered a veritable wealth of information, including the Bechamp story. From then on, my husband Julian and I decided we had to endeavor to rectify, as much as possible, a grave injustice done to a brilliant scientist. To do that, meant writing to as many international scientists and doctors as possible. . .

"Of course, to capture their interest, we had to present some sort of a case showing the relevance of the microzymian theory to modern molecular biology and genetics, bio-energetics, and even physics. If I possess any talent, I would suggest that the German philosopher Goethe quoted it as such: 'Scientific discovery consists in seeing an analogy where nobody has seen one before.'

"We realize your obvious disappointment that there are no drawings of microzymas. To photograph the glittering motile microzymas that Bechamp observed in The Kitten Experiment might be possible with modern photographic equipment.

"As for your observations of the cell wall deficient, granular, coccoid forms — they would be a 'phase' of microzymian 'vibrionen evolution' — (infinite in their variety of forms). You wrote you were constantly amazed how the bacterial isolates from diseased skin change form, species, and even classification — right before your very eyes, depending on what you 'feed' the microbes. Recall that Bechamp said 'microzymas become BY NUTRITION what they ought to become.'

"Virginia Livingston's observations of *Progenitor cryptocides* goes close to the truth, but the various stages of the cancer microbe actually demonstrate Bechamp's various stages of vibrionen evolution. However, Dr. Livingston applies this within the orbit of the Pasteurian Dogma, as many others do also. But only the pure and simple expression of the microzymian thesis can provide the answer as to 'why this is so.'

"In your book, *AIDS: THE MYSTERY AND THE SOLUTION*, you made reference to the AIDS retrovirus containing an enzyme (Bechamp's ferment) called reverse transcriptase — which allows the virus to reproduce itself backwards by transferring or transposing viral RNA into DNA. You also wrote, 'the ability to switch genetic material backward from RNA to DNA defied the long held scientific dictum that genetic transfer could only occur in one direction.'

"For some understanding of why this is so — read pages 409 to 417 of *THE BLOOD*. You will read: 'The microzymas are ORGANIZED FERMENTS, they can (under favorable circumstances) produce bacteria; under other circumstances the microzymas become builders of cellules. All organisms are created by them.'

"In short, the cell — and even the bacterium itself — can rebecome a microzyma! Thus, the microzymas (the small ferments) are seen to be both the 'beginning' as well as the 'end' of all life as we know it. Certainly, genetic material can be switched backward.

"In diseases such as cancer and AIDS, it appears that as the putrefaction of blood and tissue sets in — and 'matter' is destroyed — the microzymas undergo change and transpose into their primitive condition. Bechamp states clearly, 'The microzymas, whether in the state of bacteria or not, are sufficient to assure by putrifaction — the circulation of matter.'

"Before closing this letter, a few thoughts about the cancer microbe. Let us take leukemia for instance. We all know excessive exposure to radiation can cause leukemia. (Virus or microbe not required here.) There are countless carcinogenic agents that can lead to cancer. Vaccines can also be dangerous. We have always believed that vaccines disrupt the normal functioning of many cells, including the T-cells of the immune system. Degenerative diseases such as cancer and AIDS can be provoked as a result of all these agents.

"Once a body is in the state of disease — such as AIDS — the disease can be communicated to others — but only under certain circumstances. (Resistance factors, etc., come into play.) Bechamp did not deny the specificity of certain viral and bacterial infectious diseases. But his microzyma theory explains what

Florence Nightingale has put so eloquently. After observing the outbreak of infectious diseases among her soldier-patients in the Crimea, the famous nurse insisted — 'There are no specific diseases, only specific disease *conditions*.'

"On that note, I bring this letter to a close, thanking you once again for your patience and willingness to offer us a hearing. We hope that what is written here will prove helpful to you in your search for the truth." — (Signed) Dorothy Knafelc.

Through the kindness of my Australian contacts, I soon received a photocopy of Antoine Bechamp's *THE BLOOD AND ITS THIRD ANATOMIC ELEMENT*[1]. The book heavily details the fermentation experiments that enthralled Bechamp and Pasteur, as well as the disagreements between the two nineteenth century scientists. Without a good knowledge of biochemistry, it is a difficult book to read. Nevertheless, it contains a remarkable presentation of Bechamp's microzymian theory and his views about the blood.

In Bechamp's view, the blood is not simply a liquid but rather a living, flowing tissue. Within this tissue are three vital anatomic elements: the red cells, the white cells, and the heretofore unrecognized microzymas — the 'third anatomic element' of the blood. Bechamp deplored Pasteur's refusal to acknowledge the existence of microzymas. Without a knowledge of the nature and function of microzymas, the chemist and his followers could never understand human disease.

For a long time I mulled over Bechamp's old research and theories. Was he really the forgotten scientific genius of his age? Would his microzyma theory of disease ever replace (or complement) Pasteur's well-established germ

theory of disease? Was Pasteur's meteoric rise to world
fame more "show business" than science?

As my file on Bechamp enlarged with continuing
correspondence from down under, I started to piece
together the strange series of events that catapulted the
French professor's ideas into the twentieth century, and
into my life. The Australian connection began in the late
1950s with Archie Kalokerinos MD.

Archie was born in New South Wales, Australia, the
grandson of a Greek immigrant. After graduating from
medical school in Sydney in 1951, Archie continued his
studies in England, but he missed the beauty and
warmth of Australia, and returned in 1957. Unimpressed
with money and prestige, Archie chose to practice in the
Australian outback. He settled in the tiny town of
Collarenebri, 500 miles northwest of Sydney, in the heart
of Aboriginal country. He fell in love with the land and
the people — and stayed 17 years.

The death rate for the impoverished Aboriginals was
appalling; and bacterial, viral, and parasitic infections
were common. Most frightening were the alarming
number of "crib deaths," the sudden deaths of infants
from no apparent cause. It took years for Archie to
realize that some of these deaths were caused by the
poor nutrition of the Aboriginal children. He eventually
learned that massive infusions of Vitamin C could save
these babies. Even though the children did not show the
classic signs and symptoms of scurvy, Archie insisted
the children were deficient in Vitamin C. His medical
colleagues strongly disagreed, and they accused Archie
of causing trouble by incorrectly diagnosing Vitamin C
deficiency (scurvy) in Aboriginals.

In his book, *EVERY SECOND CHILD*, Dr. Kalokerinos writes: "Why my observations concerning vitamin

deficiencies among Aboriginals became so controversial I will never know. The situation was obvious. One could see what they ate — sugar, bread, jam and sausage — and one did not need to be an expert, or to employ teams of dieticians and chemists to perform intricate assays, in order to know what these consisted of. Yet, whenever I spoke about deficiencies, there was an uproar and I was labeled a ratbag. In itself this did not worry me, but I knew beyond any doubt that if infants were supplemented with vitamins as an emergency measure until diets could be improved, the Aboriginal infant death throughout Australia would drop by half."[2]

A team of scientists, headed by Glen Dettman, was finally sent to Collarenebri to quell Archie's Vitamin C controversy. When Glen's team completed their investigation, Archie was vindicated. The laboratory tests indeed proved the Aboriginals were deficient in Vitamin C.

In 1970 the Australian government stepped up their vaccination programs. The results were disastrous for the Aboriginal children. The infant death rate in the Northern Territory suddenly doubled. By 1971 the death rate, in some areas, was approaching 500 per 1000 infants. Archie watched "every second child" die.

Archie blamed the government's vaccine program for causing the horrendous rise in the children's mortality rate. Immunization shots might be OK for healthy children but for Aboriginals, due to their nutritional and vitamin deficiences, it was life-threatening.

In his book, Archie wrote that the authorities would line up the children for vaccinations. "There would be no examination, no taking of case histories, no checking of dietary deficiencies. Most infants would have colds. No wonder they died. Some would die within hours from acute vitamin C deficiency precipitated by the immunization. Others would suffer immunological insults and die later from 'pneumonia,' 'gastroenteritis' or 'malnutrition.' If some babies and infants survived, they would be lined up again within a month for another immunization. If some managed to survive even this, they would be lined up again. Then there would be booster shots, shots for measles, polio and even TB. Little wonder they died. The wonder is that any survived."

Vaccines are the legacy of Pasteur; and the legendary story of the little boy bitten by the rabid dog and saved from certain death by Pasteur's anti-rabies vaccine is known the world over. When I was a young boy I remember a wonderful Hollywood movie about Pasteur's life that starred Paul Muni.

Spurred on by Pasteur's vaccine miracles, the pharmaceutical industry quickly saw the commercial advantage of a vaccine or a drug for every disease caused by Pasteur's air germs. Public health officials are aware of the dangers of vaccines, but officials also know that forced vaccine programs can produce spectacular results in quelling epidemic disease. The perils of immunization are always downplayed by physicians and drug companies. In the interest of public health, physicians rarely warn parents about the severe and occasionally fatal consequences of vaccine administration.

As expected, the Australian government denied that the vaccine programs were related to the increased mortality rates in children. But vaccine experiments in animals proved that Archie was right. High doses of vitamin C in animals reversed the toxic and deadly effects of experimental vaccination.

Archie and Glen's controversial and inflammatory views on the dangers of vaccines were unpopular in the medical community; and stories of their fight against the government's forced vaccine programs in the Aboriginal communities appeared in the newspapers. The story prompted Dorothy Knafelc to write Archie and Glen, offering a scientific explanation for the vaccine deaths.

Dorothy suspected the vaccines were acting on the microzymas with disastrous results, especially if the "little ferments" were already altered by co-existent infection in the child's body, or by nutritional deficiency, or both. The followers of Pasteur and the vaccine makers knew nothing about these factors because, in their view, microzymas did not exist.

Archie and Glen were medical heretics who warned the public about the deadly effects of "life-saving vaccines." Taking Dorothy's advice, they studied Bechamp's writings and theories.

In *EVERY SECOND CHILD* Archie gives credit to Dorothy. "Knowledge is a powerful weapon and has eased the enormous responsibility that once weighed so hard upon my shoulders. For much of this I owe a debt to Dorothy Knafelc, who has worked so tirelessly on my behalf. The nature of infections and their relationships to nutrition and the environment are difficult, in fact impossible, to understand unless the errors in the Pasteurian line of thinking are pointed out. 'Germs' do not cause disease in the real sense. Something happens in the body to allow the germs to become invasive."

In August 1977 Archie and Glen were invited to lecture at the annual meeting of the International Academy of Preventive Medicine. Their controversial lecture entitled "Second Thoughts about Disease; A Controversy and Bechamp Revisited," was later published as a pamphlet by the Biological Research Institute in Victoria, Australia.

Archie and Glen spoke to a startled audience of

physicians. "Modern medicine is based on Pasteur's germ theory of disease — a specific disease and a specific vaccine gives specific protection. Shades of doubt concerning the validity of this dogma were seen when it was observed that some Aboriginal children did not get protection and, in fact, died when vaccines were administered. . .

"One of the great dangers of Pasteur's 'germ theory' is that it is a part truth! We would like to believe that we have presented evidence in this paper to raise valid questions concerning Pasteur's 'germ theory.' We realize that orthodox science may explain some of the questions we have raised; but would it be so outrageous to suggest that we also re-examine Bechamp's hypothesis in the light of today's knowledge of pleomorphic microorganisms, enzymes, RNA-DNA, and assorted unexplainable phenomena observed generally in the world of microorganisms. . .

"Hopefully there may be others among you who will be motivated to examine these issues and launch serious research into this lost chapter in the history of microbiology. Such an investigation, we feel, will cause one of the biggest medical upsets of the century, and we welcome inquiries from those who decide to contribute to bringing the light of understanding to this important subject."[3]

Thus, a trio of Australians composed of a physician, a microbiologist, and a scholarly housewife who discovered Bechamp's work in the British Museum, continue to inform scientists about the long-forgotten French Professor.

In 1988 John West of Queensland, Australia, published *THE AIDS TIME BOMB*,[4] a book implicating monkey virus-contaminated vaccines as the cause of the AIDS

outbreak. John is also an outspoken advocate of
Bechamp. In his book he wrote, "The only subjects
worthy of serious study are sex, death, and microzymas."
His company, Veritas Press, has also reissued Bechamp's
*THE BLOOD AND ITS THIRD ANATOMICAL
ELEMENT*[5].

When I completed my investigation of Bechamp, I had a
deeper understanding of the possible origin of the
microbes I had studied in scleroderma and cancer and
AIDS. In medical school I was taught that bacteria and
viruses always come from outside the body, never from
within as Antoine Bechamp and Edgar Cayce suggested.
As a student I briefly wondered how a chemist could
have become "the father of modern medicine." But like
most doctors I never questioned established dogma. The
reason Pasteur was correct was because all the doctors
and the scientists believed he was correct — and that
was that!
    I felt a strange affinity for Bechamp and his work. We
had both seen microbes where there weren't supposed to
be any. I had seen them in a variety of diseases, and
even in "normal" tissue. . . and so did Bechamp. I
observed microbes change form and species and classification in the laboratory, even though they weren't
supposed to. Bechamp was right, and the chemist was
wrong. I suspected the cancer microbe could originate
from within the tissue cells of the body; and so did
Bechamp. But Pasteur never saw microzymas and the
cancer microbe, and all Pasteur's microbes came from
the "outside."
    Virginia had initially opened my mind to the idea that
the cancer microbe could arise from within the cell, but
she also believed that cancer microbes came from

without. That was why she instructed her patients carefully about diet. She urged them to avoid infected meats, and chicken, and dairy products. And Virginia produced cancer by injecting cancer microbes into animals, just like Robert Koch produced TB in animals.

The more I studied the microbiology of cancer, the more difficult it was to reconcile all my findings in terms of traditional microbiology. The cancer microbe could never be classified because it broke all the established rules of biology. It was a virus, a granule, a bacterium, a yeast, a fungus, and a parasite that none of the cancer experts could see.

Bechamp made sense of the cancer microbe because he knew that all the various forms of the cancer microbe were infinite expressions of the transformed and diseased microzymas! I finally understood why Pasteur sought to destroy Bechamp. Pasteur's "germ theory" gave birth to the science of microbiology; Bechamp sought to abort the new science of microbiology by looking deeper into the cellular "microzymian" origin of disease.

My study of Bechamp had shattered the icon of Pasteur. The chemist made germs respectable and he was a genius at popularizing microbes as a cause of human disease. He gave the world "pasteurization," a monumental achievement. But he also put medical science on the wrong track. Pasteur's dogma transformed the art and science of medicine into a multibillion dollar biotechnical business in search of a perfect pill and a perfect vaccine to cure man of all his ills.

In the process the physicians were blinded. They could not see or comprehend the microzymas and the forces that pervaded and propelled all life. And they did not understand that derangement of this life force could lead to cancer, degenerative disease, and death.

As Bechamp lay dying in Paris, he mulled over his life. At age ninety-two, he had outlived his wife and all his children. No one could console him. Yet he took pride in his accomplishments as a scientist and a physician and a teacher. He had relentlessly studied the microzymas — the little ferments that brilliantly directed the life of the cell.

He had led a quiet family life, unconcerned with personal glory and fame. Yes, he had fought bitterly with Pasteur, but only to defend the existence of his precious microzymas. He was uncomfortable bickering with Pasteur; it was not part of his nature. He was born under the Venus-ruled sign of Libra, the sign of balance and harmony. It was these qualities that so endeared him to the little bodies he avidly studied in the cells. He had uncovered the sparks of life that lay hidden within the microzymas. He sensed the delicate balance and the necessary harmony that were the essential ingredients for healthy and never-ending life.

As Bechamp was laid to rest, an eleven year-old farmboy played in the fields, a thousand miles to the east of Paris, in the vast expanse of the Austro-Hungarian Empire. The boy, Wilhelm Reich, was born under the powerful Mars-ruled sign of Aries — the sign of the ego, the pioneer, and the male force. Unlike Bechamp, he would take the backseat to no one; and he would pay dearly for it.

Bechamp had discovered an indestructible force that pervaded every living cell. The boy would soon recognize the force in his loins. As a physician, he would scientifically demonstrate the force in the erogenous zones, and then in the tumors of cancer, and finally within every living and non-living object on the planet.

Bechamp and Reich found a new, god-like force of nature that blurred the boundary between life and death. Their discoveries were among the greatest the world had ever known. But by the end of the twentieth century, there were few people who realized what had been accomplished.

References:

1. **Bechamp A**: *The Blood and its Third Anatomic Element*. John Ouseley Ltd, London, England, 1912.

2. **Kalokerinos, A**: *Every Second Child*. Keats Publishing Co., New Canaan, Connecticut, 1981.

3. **Kalokerinos A, Dettman G**: Second thoughts about disease; A controversy and Bechamp revisited, J Intl Acad Preventive Medicine 4(1), July 1977.

4. **West J**: *The AIDS Time Bomb*. Veritas Press, Bundaberg, Queensland, Australia, 1988.

5. **Bechamp A**: *The Blood and its Third Anatomic Element*. (Available from Veritas Press, Box 1653 GPO, Bundaberg, Queensland, Australia, 4670).

CHAPTER ELEVEN

Reich's Bions

In my struggle to uncover the secrets of the cancer microbe I never dreamed I would become enmeshed in the strange world of Wilhelm Reich. For two decades I studied the work of scientists who had linked bacteria to cancer. Never did I find a reference to Reich's important experiments with the deadly "T-bacilli" that he discovered in cancer. Nor did Virginia or Eleanor ever mention his work. Yet they were all scientific contemporaries who lived in the New York City area in the 1940s and 50s.

After studying Reich, I became convinced that his cancer theories, along with Virginia and Eleanor's cancer microbe work, comprised the most logical scientific explanation not only for the origin of cancer, but for the origin of life itself.

I understood why scientists were silent about Reich's cancer research. His discoveries were deemed dangerous to society, and his story was a messy one, best eliminated from the annals of modern medical history. Reich's radical cancer experiments and theories remain embarrassments which bear the seal of official disapproval. As a result of the scientific inquisition against him, Reich's stupendous cancer discoveries seem destined for obscurity along with Bechamp's microzymas.

A doctor friend advised me not to mention Reich in my writings: he was too controversial and too crazy. Referring to Reich would only detract from my credibility as a researcher. But it was impossible to dismiss Reich's cancer microbe research. When *AIDS: THE*

MYSTERY AND THE SOLUTION was published in 1984, I included Reich as one of the foremost scientists in cancer microbiology[1].

In 1982, Lorraine Rosenthal of the Cancer Control Society first told me about Wilhelm Reich. Her mother had worked in his laboratory in Maine in the 1950s. Lorraine was sure Reich's cancer work was related to my cancer microbe research, and she recommended that I read two of Reich's books available at the CCS bookstore.

Reich's two most revolutionary books, *THE BION EXPERIMENTS ON THE ORIGIN OF LIFE* (1938)[2] and *THE CANCER BIOPATHY* (1948)[3], contain the details of his highly controversial biologic experiments and scientific theories. These two volumes provide valuable and fascinating insights into the origin of the cancer cell and the significance of cancer "T" bacteria.

During his life, Reich was portrayed as a mad psychiatrist and scientist who advocated "free love," abortion, communism, and a multitude of other perversions. The medical establishment regarded him as a quack, who tried to dupe the public into believing he had a cure for cancer. Under public pressure, the U.S. government finally took legal action to suppress Reich and the new science he was proclaiming. The closing years of his life were filled with tragedy. Persecuted and hounded by the government, he was finally sacrificed on the altar of science.

Who was Wilhelm Reich, and why was he condemned for his beliefs? Was he merely a crack-pot psychiatrist? Or was he one of the greatest scientific geniuses of the twentieth century?

Reich was born March 24, 1897, in a small farm

community in Bukovina at the eastern edge of the Austro-Hungarian Empire. At age twelve, his childhood was shattered by his mother's suicide. Provoked by marital unhappiness and infidelity, despondency, and beatings by her husband, she swallowed a kitchen poison. The young Reich watched her die a slow, agonizing death. Reich's father died of tuberculosis in 1914; and twelve years later, Reich's only brother also died of TB. Reich himself briefly came down with the disease in 1927. Further details of Reich's early life can be found in the recently published, *PASSION OF YOUTH: AN AUTOBIOGRAPHY*[4].

Orphaned at age 17, Reich entered the Austrian army and experienced the brutality of World War 1 and the ensuing break-up of the Austro-Hungarian Empire; and the ceding of his homeland, Bukovina, to Romania. After the war he resumed his studies in Vienna and entered medical school. Reich was a brilliant student who developed a strong liking for the new specialty of psychiatry. At age twenty-three, he became one of Sigmund Freud's prized associates and began private practice as an analytic psychiatrist.

Reich was consumed by the study of sexuality and its effect on the psyche. Drawing upon his own sexual feelings and experiences, as well as those of his patients, he espoused controversial sexual theories that stunned his colleagues. Using novel experimental methods he examined, analysed, and even measured various aspects of physical lovemaking. The young psychiatrist concluded that the ability to love was dependent on one's physical ability to make love with "orgastic potency." Reich coined this term to denote a kind of superlovemaking in which the mental, physical, and emotional aspects of sexuality were all functioning at a high level.

Reich dissected human sexuality the way anatomists dissected the body. Experimenting with electrical stimulation of erogenous zones, he showed that sexual feelings like touch, pleasure, and pain could be measured in the laboratory. Reich was a pioneer in the scientific study and analysis of human sexuality.

The physiologic process of erection of the male penis provided a formula for Reich's greatest scientific discoveries. Before male orgasm, Reich noted that four distinct and separate processes had to take place physiologically. First is the necessary psychosexual build-up or "tension." Second, the "charge" that accompanies tumescence of the penis, which Reich measured electrically. Third, the electrical "discharge" at the moment of orgasm. And fourth, the final "relaxation" of the penis.

Reich observed these four essential stages (tension, build-up, discharge, and relaxation) in all aspects of life that he examined. In sex, he discovered an energy and a force that was unique to life. Reich believed this force pervaded all nature. He named this force "orgone energy."

With the professional support of Sigmund Freud, Reich quickly rose to the highest ranks of academia. His classic book, *CHARACTER ANALYSIS* (1933), recounts his original and brilliant contributions to psychiatry. Foremost is Reich's novel concept of "body armoring."

Through the teachings of the early twentieth century psychiatrists, we now readily accept the concept that people react to the stresses and strains of life by externalizing or internalizing their emotional energy. However, other psychiatric teachings and theories are more controversial. For example, Freud shocked the public by suggesting that children were sexual, and by popularizing the Oedipus-complex theory (the child wanting to marry the parent of the opposite sex, and killing the parent of the same sex). According to Freud and other psychiatrists, these childhood sexual conflicts form the basis of neurotic behavior in adulthood.

Reich discovered that unreleased psychosexual energy could produce actual physical "blocks" within the muscles and organs of the body. These blocks are the "armor" which prevent the release of this blocked sexual energy. The orgasm, along with the convulsive body spasms which accompany orgasm, is the mechanism through which this "orgone energy" is released.

Reich believed a healthy and loving sex life was everyone's right. In fact, a good sex life was absolutely necessary for the proper functioning of the body. He stressed that the social and political ills of the world stemmed largely from society's repression of sexuality. This repression leads to unhappiness, depression, and the inability to express joyous sexual love. For countless numbers of people the sexual energy is blocked because of personal body armoring. As a result of this armoring, such people often fall victim to various aspects of the "emotional plague."

In *THE FUNCTION OF THE ORGASM* (1942) Reich wrote: "Mental illness is a result of a disturbance in the natural capacity for love. In the case of orgastic impotence, from which a vast majority of humans are suffering, biological energy is dammed up, thus becoming the source of all kinds of irrational behavior. The cure of the psychic disturbances requires in the first place the establishment of the natural capacity for love. It depends as much upon social as upon psychic conditions. Antisocial behavior springs from secondary drives which owe their existence to the suppression of natural sexuality."[5]

In his practice of analytic psychiatry, Reich broke with tradition. Instead of sitting passively, notebook in hand while his patients talked, Reich took an active role in the therapy. He frequently touched his patients, felt their chests for breathing, and repositioned their bodies. Sometimes he badgered and goaded them to physical action. In order to observe their body response during analysis, Reich sometimes insisted that all or part of the clothing be removed. Men were often reduced to shorts; women to bra and panties. Reich's colleagues publicly protested against these unorthodox and radical psychiatric practices. His most vociferous opponents accused him of immorality.

The post-World War I period was a time of intense political and social unrest, particularly in Austria and Germany. As a young man in Vienna during the 1920s and 30s, Reich was exceedingly active in political movements for social reform. Disliking the anti-sexual right-wing conservatives and repelled by the fanaticism of the fascists, he migrated to Marxism. In the years following the Russian revolution, Reich admired the Soviet dream of a better world for the common masses. The communists were also proclaiming a sexual freedom that was in marked contrast to the party ideology of the Christian right-wing conservatives and the fascists. In 1927 Reich joined the Communist Party, and became one of its leading advocates in promoting sexual reform for the masses.

Although Reich was a noted sex expert, his expertise did not carry over to the state of matrimony. In 1922 he wed Annie Pink, a psychiatrist. Their first child, Eva, was born in 1924. A second daughter was born in 1928. The marriage was chaotic. Reich's revolutionary ideas about sexual relationships undoubtedly contributed to the marital discord. No matter how hard he tried, it was impossible for Reich to conform to marital conventions. The outspoken Reich even went so far as to propose that a series of romantic relationships ("serial monogamy") was a better alternative to marriage.

In *THE FUNCTION OF THE ORGASM* (1927) he declared: "Marriage is only one of the many issues where social scientists go astray, especially since they fail to see marriage for what it really is — a sexual union, based primarily on genital love. They prefer to ignore that fact and merely view it as an economic union or means to perpetuate the human race. Actually very few people marry just for money or to have children; marriages of today really limit peoples' freedom and may lead to economic deprivation."[6]

For professional, political, and social reasons, Reich moved his analytic practice to Berlin in 1930. He joined the German Communist Party, convinced that the sexual freedoms of Marxism would liberate the common man and foster his mental health. As a spokesman for the Party, Reich publicly advocated free contraceptives, birth control, abortion on demand, and sex education in schools.

For Reich and Germany, 1933 was an eventful year. Reich's marriage was on the rocks, and he was already involved in another passionate love relationship. The German communists were becoming increasingly disenchanted with the controversial Reich. The communists were trying to win public confidence, not destroy it by Reich's outrageous ideas on sexual-political matters. Finally, the Party expelled Reich.

To make matters worse, he was in a career crisis. In the beginning the psychiatric establishment accepted him because of his close association with Freud. But as Reich's psychiatric writings and his political left-wing activities became progressively more out of tune with Freud's ideas, his professional relationship with his colleagues cooled. Political pressure was put on the Psychoanalytic Association to get rid of Reich and his radical ideas and politics. In a supreme blow to Reich's career, the Association revoked his membership.

All this personal turbulence was compounded by the rise of Hitler and Nazism. In January 1933 Hitler became Chancellor of Germany. In March, Reich's sexual-political writings were attacked in the Nazi press. He was damned as a radical psychiatrist, an anti-Nazi communist, a womanizer, and a Jew. Berlin was no longer safe for Reich. Disguised as a tourist on a ski trip to Austria, he luckily got out of the city by the skin of his teeth[7].

Returning to Vienna, Reich realized that his politics and his unorthodox brand of psychiatry were no longer welcome. He emigrated to Denmark but soon became embroiled in disputes with the Danish communists, which forced his departure. From there, he relocated to Sweden, but was again harassed by the authorities. Finally, through the help of Norwegian colleagues, he secured residence in Oslo.

By 1934, Reich's divorce was finalized. Fortunately, Annie and the children escaped the Nazis and were resettled in Austria. Reich was madly in love with Elsa Lindenberg, who followed him in his exodus to Austria, Denmark, Sweden, and finally to Norway. Now through the kind assistance of his Norwegian friends, he had a new laboratory and enough money to continue his research.

Reich's work in Norway was quite different from what

it had been previously. To help pay bills, he continued practicing as an analytic psychiatrist, but now his first love was orgone research. Years earlier he had focused on the orgasm and its implications. The orgasm contained the key to the life force: the four-step principle of tension, charge, discharge and relaxation. Now he was determined to master all the secrets of this new force he had discovered.

Reich began his experiments simply. His previous experiments with electrical stimulation of the skin cells of the erogenous zones had taught him that these sexual areas carried an unusual electric charge. He decided to experiment with the smallest form of cell life known to man: the so-called "protozoa."

Protozoa are life forms composed of only one cell. In Reich's time, one form of protozoa known as the amoeba (plural: amoebae) was considered the most primitive form of animal life. A 1950s textbook explained: "An amoeba appears as simple as a fully developed organism can be, and it is famous on that account. It has become a living symbol of the primitive, as in the common expression 'from amoeba to man,' although it is improbable that anything quite like an amoeba ever did figure in our ancestry.'[8] Currently, scientific opinion has changed: the one-cell protozoa and amoebae are now classified as "neither plants nor animals but belong instead to a separate kingdom."[9]

For the past several centuries biologists have known that it is possible to grow amoebae by taking hay (semi-dry grass) and immersing it in water. After about two weeks, amoebae usually appear in the hay-water infusion.

Reich hadn't studied microbiology for years. Arriving

at the Oslo Botanical Institute to pick up the flask
containing the hay-water mixture from which the
amoebae would grow, Reich naively asked the lab
instructor, "Where do the amoebae come from?" The
instructor, glancing disdainfully at Reich in disbelief,
replied, "From the germs in the air, of course."

Reich's lab was blessed with the finest microscopes
money could buy. Ordinary microscopes magnify about
1000 times, but Reich owned powerful microscopes that
could magnify 2000-3000 times, or even higher. This
higher magnification (above 1000x) proved essential for
Reich's discoveries.

Reich established a primary rule for scientific work:
"Do not automatically believe in anything; convince
yourself of something by observing it with your own eyes
and, having perceived a fact, do not lose sight of it
again until it has been fully explained."[3]

Reich (in typically impatient Aries fashion) saw no
reason to wait two weeks for the amoebae to appear in
the hay-water infusion. Instead, he observed the
immersed blades of grass every day. After several days,
he noticed the changes in the cells of the grass as they
degenerated and decomposed in the water. Little
"vesicular" bubbly swellings appeared in the grass cells.
At the edges of the blades of grass Reich saw the tiny
vesicles breaking out of the cells and detaching themselves into the water. When two weeks passed, the
amoebae formed in the water, just as the instructor
predicted. But to Reich's keen eye, the one-celled
amoebae looked strikingly similar in size and shape to
the vesicular swellings that had formed inside the cells
and had broken away into the water.

Reich thought: "The living vesicular ('honeycomb')
plasma of the amoeba must be very closely related to

the vesicular structure of the disintegrated plants. Could it be possible that an amoeba or other protozoan with a similar vesicular structure is nothing more that a cluster of vesicles enclosed and shaped by a membrane?"[3]

Reich marveled at the squirming amoebae. They were seemingly simple structureless blobs. Yet, they were also exceedingly complex life forms containing a nucleus and cytoplasm filled with barely visible granules. The protozoa ate, digested, contracted, expelled, and multiplied. He playfully applied a small electric current and watched the protozoa contract and elongate.

During the years 1934-1937, Reich was totally absorbed in his experiments on the origin of life. His preparations consisted of infusions of various substances: grass, beach sand, earth, coal, iron filings, animal tissue, and other substances. He tested various combinations and added potassium, gelatin, and other biochemicals to the mixtures. Boiling the preparations resulted in a marked increase in the number of "vesicles" that could be cultured.

After much experimentation, Reich concluded that the cultured vesicles were intermediate "transitional" forms, which were "midway between life and non-life." "Dead" inorganic substances (such as sand, earth, and coal) gave birth to vesicles which pulsed with life. Reich named these energetic vesicles "bions." And he suspected bions were a heretofore unrecognized elementary stage of life.

Then Reich did a strange thing with his boiled bion cultures. After cooling, he poured some of the boiled material onto laboratory nutrient culture media designed to grow ordinary bacteria. An unbelievable phenomenon resulted: the boiled bion cultures gave birth to peculiar-looking bacteria, and amoebae!

Reich had to be sure these microbes were not

contaminating germs from the air or from improperly sterilized laboratory culture media. To eliminate these two possible sources of contamination, he heated his bion cultures to the intense, flaming, glowing temperatures of incandescence (1500 degrees centigrade). He repeatedly sterilized his laboratory culture media by autoclaving it at a high temperature (180 degrees centigrade) and pressure. No known bacteria or any other life form could possibly survive at such a high temperature and pressure. He deliberately exposed his bion cultures to the "germs in the air," but the cultures never became contaminated with the kind of microbes that grew in his sterilized bion cultures.

Despite all these attempts at sterilizing everything in the experiment, the superheated "dead" bion mixtures still gave rise to bacteria and pulsating amoebae in the nutrient media. Like Antoine Bechamp, Wilhelm Reich discovered an indestructible life force of nature that defied death. Reich finally concluded: Bions are preliminary stages of life; they are transitional forms from the inorganic and non-motile — to the organic, motile, and culturable state.

When Reich's *THE BION EXPERIMENTS* was published in Oslo in 1938, the book created a furor. He was accused of attacking the sacred dogma of science by attempting to overthrow a half-century of modern medical progress. Reich had audaciously refuted the "germ theory" teachings of Louis Pasteur, and he would pay dearly for this transgression.

In some ways, Reich was naive; he simply could not understand the uproar surrounding his bion experiments. But his critics latched onto one paragraph in the Bion book that intimated Reich might have inadvertently found a cancer cure. Reich had written that preliminary studies showed bion-like structures that could be cultured from human blood. According to Reich, "bion research proved particularly fruitful for an understanding of cancer."

The scientific and lay press attacked him unmercifully, claiming the "Jew pornographer" was tinkering with life and promoting a quack cancer cure. His enemies called for the immediate expulsion of this mad foreigner from Norway[7].

Controversy followed Reich like smoke follows fire, but the attacks on his scientific credibility had a curious effect. Instead of discouraging him, the attacks lured him deeper and deeper into orgone research. In spite of the harassment Reich was determined to prove, beyond doubt, the reality of the new life energy forms he had discovered in his experiments.

Important scientific discoveries sometimes happen by accident. A great scientist can recognize the importance of such an event; and great scientists are rare. Even rarer are scientists who have the intuition, the foresight, and the fortitude to pursue a great discovery to its logical scientific conclusion. It was these essential characteristics that made Reich the brilliant scientist that he was.

The unfair accusations surrounding the publication of *THE BIONS EXPERIMENTS* goaded Reich into trying to solve the mystery of cancer. Weeks earlier he had placed some sterile cancer tissue (provided by the surgeons at the local hospital) into flasks containing liquid nutrient broth. Now, in his anger, he scurried around the lab to retrieve the bottles. To his astonishment, "all these cultures showed a green-blue coloration. Taking material from the margin, (Reich) inoculated a new agar plate and saw, for the first time, the T-bacilli, the discovery of which would help break down the mystery surrounding the cancer problem."[3]

The finding of bacteria in cancer filled Reich with a curious mixture of fear and awe. With fear, because he knew that solving the secrets of cancer would be a Herculean task, further antagonizing the medical establishment against him. With awe, because he intuitively knew these bacilli were involved in the agonizing cancer deaths that affected countless millions. After much study Reich named his newly-discovered cancer microbes "T" bacilli, after the German word "tod," meaning death.

The exploration of the bions and the T-bacilli became Reich's personal mission. In this effort he was essentially alone because there were few scientists who could even remotely understand the implications of the bion work. But Reich possessed a rare, God-given gift. He was given the opportunity and the key to unlock nature's greatest secret. He had no choice. He was compelled to continue the work that he was destined to accomplish.

The years 1934-1937 in Norway were Reich's happiest. The bion work was exceedingly productive; and he was deeply in love with Elsa Lindenberg.

In August 1938, Hitler annexed Austria. Miraculously, Annie and the children had emigrated to America the month before. Unlike most Norwegians, Reich correctly predicted that Hitler would eventually invade Norway, just as he had invaded Austria.

Reich's lingering presence in Norway increasingly angered the authorities. The newspaper attacks against Reich were unrelenting, and there were few people he could turn to for support and encouragement. Aggravated by depression and bouts of jealously and pettiness, his relationship with Elsa cooled. As Norwegian officials put increasing pressure on him to leave the country, an American colleague strongly urged Reich to emigrate to the United States.

In August 1939, on the last boat to leave Norway before the war, Reich left for America. Half-heartedly he had asked Elsa to come, but their tempestuous love affair was over, and beyond repair. Reich never saw her again.

By this time Reich was completely disillusioned with the communists and their false promises and their perversion of Marx's humanitarian ideals. When the Russians joined with the Nazis to sever Poland, he saw the communists for what they truly were. Never again would their philosophy interest him, and he became an ardent anti-communist.

When he embarked for America, Wilhelm Reich was no longer young. He was 42 years old and he would again be a stranger in a strange land.

Arriving in New York in August 1939, he rented a house in Forest Hills, Long Island. Soon he began a new love affair with Ilse Ollendorff, who was extremely helpful in assisting Reich with his research. They married in 1946 and Ilse bore him a son, Peter.

The cancer work, which began with the discovery of T-bacilli in 1937, continued with a frenzy. The T-bacilli proved to be the key to the origin of cancer. Reich's experiments showed that all life contains orgone energy. When the orgone energy diminishes in the cells, either through injury or aging, the cells undergo a death process that Reich termed "bionous degeneration." As a consequence of decreased cellular orgone energy and bionous degeneration, the deadly T-bacilli begin to form in the cells.

Reich microscopically examined various types of cancer. Unlike most scientists, he carefully studied the cancer cells in the living, unstained state. At magnifications of 2000x, he discovered the T-bacilli in the cancer tumors. Cultures of T-bacilli injected into mice caused inflammation and death from cancer.

The T-bacilli that formed in the cells provoked a reaction in the tissues that resulted in the formation of vesicular swellings. Microscopically, these vesicles gave off a bluish glow. Reich called them "blue PA bions" because they resembled the clumped "PAcket" bions that were experimentally produced when he heated substances (such as grass and coal) to high temperatures.

In degenerating cancerous tissue, the blue PA bions seriously affect the orgone energy of the cells. As a result of this bion activity, the usual pentagonal shape of the cells softens into round forms; and granules appear in the cells. Granules also appear in the spaces between the cells and spread into the surrounding tissue. The cells eventually clump together and form club-shaped and spindly-shaped cells characteristic of typical cancer cells. In cancer tumors artificially produced in animals, Reich observed the animals' cancer cells transform into monster cells that greatly resembled tiny protozoa and amoebae![7] In mouse experiments, Reich injected blue bions into the tissue and observed the development of actual protozoa.

These cancerous changes that Reich induced were similar to what occurred in the death process when cut blades of grass were immersed in water. First the tissue cells swelled and formed vesicles; and eventually the vesicles transformed into protozoa.

Reich found that cancer cells have less orgone energy than normal, healthy cells. As the energy-depleted cancer cells break down and degenerate into T-bacilli, putrifaction of the body occurs. It is the overwhelming (and hidden) infection with T-bacilli and the massive breakdown of cancer tissue that causes most deaths from cancer. Cancer is literally death in the living body.

T-bacilli are always involved in precancerous conditions. However, once the actual cancer cells develop, the T-bacilli are no longer essential for the cancer process to continue. As the cancer cells begin to grow and multiply, the cancerous process becomes self-replicating.

Reich discovered T-bacilli not only in the cancer tumors, but also in the blood, the body fluids, and the excreta of cancer patients. He originally thought that the T-bacillus was the specific infectious agent of cancer. BUT THESE CANCER MICROBES WERE EVENTUALLY FOUND IN PERSONS WITH OTHER DISEASES — AND REICH ALSO OBSERVED THE T-BACILLI IN THE BLOOD AND EXCRETA OF NORMAL HEALTHY PEOPLE!

However, there was a difference between the blood of cancer patients and the blood of healthy people. The blood of cancer patients produced T-bacilli easily and quickly. In contrast, normal blood produced T-bacilli slowly. Reich concluded "the disposition to cancer is therefore determined by the biological resistance of the blood and the tissues to putrefaction. This biological resistance, in turn, is itself determined by the orgone energy content of the blood and the tissues, which is to say, by the organotic potency of the organism."[3]

Why can't pathologists and cancer experts understand Reich's work? One possible explanation is that they routinely study stain "dead" tissue at ordinary magnifi-

cations of 1000x. Reich studied "live" tissue, unaltered
by the physical and chemical processes required for
regular histologic preparation and tissue staining.
Neither the T-bacilli, nor the vesicular blue bions, nor
the protozoal-like cancer cells can be observed with
clarity unless microscopic magnifications of 2000-3000x
are employed. Furthermore, physicians are stuck with
the germ theory of Pasteur. Pathologists, oncologists,
and virologists all seek an external, "exogenous"
infectious viral agent in cancer. The idea of cancer
microbes originating internally within the cells is heresy.
Present-day scientists follow the teachings of Pasteur,
who argued that all microbial life originated millions of
years ago. Reich's experiments showed that microbial
life is always originating anew; and his research
indicated that the microbe of cancer originated within
us — and not from the air, as Pasteur preached.

In January 1939, Reich noted biological energy radiating
from a beach sand bion culture. The radiation seeped
from the glass bottle and pervaded his laboratory. The
following year he learned to bind this energy in a box
called the "orgone accumulator."

Ever since he first studied the energy principles of the
male erection and the orgasm, Reich followed his
scientific hunches that led him to discover a new energy
that gave the planet life.

He had strayed far from the psychiatric couch where
his patients were analysed in their underwear, or nude.
Reich was a revolutionary, and like many revolutionaries
he made powerful enemies.

During the next decade of the 1940s, his enemies
waited patiently for a chance to rid the world of this
crazy scientist and his cancer box.

Eventually they succeeded.

———————

References:

1. **Cantwell AR Jr**: *AIDS, The Mystery and the Solution*. Aries Rising Press, Los Angeles, 1984.

2. **Reich W**: *The Bion Experiments on the Origin of Life*. Ferrar, Straus and Giroux, New York, 1979.

3. **Reich W**: *The Cancer Biopathy*. Ferrar, Straus and Giroux, New York, 1973.

4. **Reich W**: *Passion of Youth; An Autobiography, 1897-1922*. Ferrar, Straus and Giroux, New York, 1988.

5. **Reich W**: *The Function of the Orgasm*. Introductory Survey, pp xxvi-xxviii, Orgone Institute Press, New York, 1942.

6. **Reich W**: The function of the orgasm (Part xi). Journal of Orgonomy 18: 143-154, 1984. (Organomic Publications, PO Box 490, Princeton, NJ 08542).

7. **Boadella D**: *Wilhelm Reich: The Evolution of His Work*. Vision Press, Chicago, 1973.

8. **Pelczar MJ Jr, Reid RD**: *Microbiology* (Ed 2). McGraw-Hill Book Co, New York, 1958.

9. **Volk WA, Wheeler MF**: *Microbiology* (Ed 4). JB Lippincott Co, Philadelphia, 1980.

CHAPTER TWELVE

Reich's Orgone Energy

Reich's early years in America were comparatively quiet compared to his turbulent years in Europe, but his biomedical activities did not go unnoticed by the authorities. In December 1941, under the guise of subversive activity, the FBI arrested Reich and detained him at Ellis Island for three weeks. The exact reasons for the arrest were never made clear, but the harrowing experience further embittered Reich against his real and imagined enemies.

In America, Reich feverishly continued his orgone experiments that began with his accidental discovery of orgone radiation in a sand bion culture in his Oslo laboratory. The radiation was initially detected during frequent microscopic examinations of a sand bion culture. After many days of peering into the eyepiece of the monocular microscope, Reich's right eye became inflamed. He suspected his eye problem might be caused by radiation coming from the sand bions (later called "sand packet" or SAPA bions). Carefully holding the bion culture tube in his hand, he felt a slight stinging sensation. Tests for regular radiation were negative. However, an electroscope detected a charge on the rubber gloves Reich used in handling the bion cultures.

Reich and his laboratory co-workers frequently experienced headaches, irritability, and other unpleasant psychological and physical effects when working with certain radioactive bion cultures. When the lab was darkened Reich detected strange, eerie blue-grey lights coming from the tubes and flasks containing the radioactive cultures. Photographic plates brought into the lab became foggy when exposed to the bion radiation.

Reich theorized the beach sand had absorbed considerable quantities of radiation from the sun. When the sand was experimentally heated to incandescence (1,500 degrees Centigrade) Reich believed the solar radiation energy contained within the sand was released into the laboratory. Whatever the precise reason, there was no doubt that orgone radiation was real. From now on, the bion cultures had to be handled with extreme care and precaution. In July 1940, Reich discovered orgone energy in the atmosphere.

In order to study the effects of this orgone radiation, Reich designed a box to house and concentrate this energy. The box was constructed with metal walls on the inside and organic material on the outside. Later, larger boxes were built to house lab animals. Still larger boxes were constructed in which a person could sit comfortably. Reich was interested in determining the effect of atmospheric orgone energy on humans, particularly persons with far-advanced and incurable forms of cancer.

It was this so-called "orgone accumulator box" and its use in human cancer experimentation that caused the Federal Drug Administration (FDA) to begin an intensive investigation of Reich's scientific activities in the late 1940s. There were all sorts of rumors and allegations concerning the box. The accumulator was widely regarded as a "sex box" which induced uncontrollable erections and stirred up intense and immoral sexual passions. As a result of this notoriety, physicians who were associated with Reich were harassed and intimidated by the authorities. Condemnatory articles in the professional and the lay press added fuel to the fire by alluding to Reich's mental problems and his sex-tinged research.

In the early 1940s Reich bought a summer house and acreage in Maine. He dearly loved the clean air, the clarity of the atmosphere, and the peacefulness of the place. Eventually he built a research lab on the site, which he named Orgonon. In 1950 he moved permanently to Orgonon. He was fifty-three years old, and tired of the stress of his psychoanalytic practice. His only desire was to devote his remaining years to orgone research.

At Orgonon, a dangerous experiment began. Reich was deeply concerned with the planetary dangers unleashed by atomic warfare at Hiroshima and Nagasaki. In the early 1950s it was feared that the Korean War might provoke another nuclear holocaust. Reich believed orgone energy could be harnessed as a possible antidote for nuclear radiation. He began testing the effects of orgone energy (OR) on nuclear energy (NR); and named the experiment "Oranur."

During the Oranur experiment, radioactive radium was brought into Reich's lab and housed in a special room containing orgone energy. The slow mixing of the two energies produced a nuclear chain reaction which had devastating consequences. As a result of this nuclear accident, Reich learned that nuclear energy drastically changed orgone energy — converting it it into "deadly orgone energy" (DOR). This laboratory accident seriously affected the physical, mental, and emotional health of Reich and his co-workers. It also necessitated a complete shut down of the lab until the dangerous radiation levels cleared.

Reich's daughter, Eva, almost died in the mishap. Eva had been estranged from her father for years, but after finishing medical school, she joined him at Orgonon to help with the Oranur experiment. The stressful changes wrought by Oranur, and the increasing harassment by the FDA, put Reich under great pressure. He was never quite the same again.

The Oranur experiment undoubtedly contributed to Reich's worsening relationship with Ilse. Despite the happiness that the birth of Peter had brought Reich, his marriage became more and more stormy. He tormented Ilse with accusations of infidelity, and was physically abusive to her. Few people understood the clinical nature of feelings and emotions better than Reich; and yet, he could be cruel, unyielding, and insanely jealous in his love relationships. He preached sexual freedom for all but he practiced a sexual double standard in marriage that allowed him to be unfaithful, but never his mate.

While Reich was immersed in the problems of Oranur, Ilse developed uterine cancer. She was convinced her cancer was connected with the radiation experiments at Orgonon. While Ilse convalesced from surgery, Reich cruelly filed for divorce. When the divorce finalized in September 1951, he began another relationship. The following month he suffered a major heart attack.

According to David Boadella's biography of Reich, "The Oranur experiment had exposed Reich and all those who worked with him to severe strains. The remainder of his life was to be devoted to working on the many problems that the atmospheric chain reaction provoked by Oranur opened up, and it was particularly unfortunate for Reich that just at the time when he was struggling to cope with the dislocation to the normal research activities of his Institute, he should become the victim of a sustained campaign to belittle, discredit and attack his work on many fronts."[1]

Despite constant attacks by the FDA, Reich pursued his experiments undaunted. He built a "cloud buster" in order to affect the orgone energy in the atmosphere. He induced rain by forcing clouds to form and disperse. Like a god, he began to control the forces of nature, as no one before him had ever done.

Reich was convinced the scientific world would recognize the value of his work and would appreciate the great benefit orgone energy could bring mankind. Long before such subjects were popular, Reich was concerned about toxic waste, nuclear energy, and planetary pollution; he knew their detrimental and damaging effects on the atmospheric orgone energy. He was sure the FDA would never destroy his research which held so much promise for the planet and its healing. Reich had implicit faith in the fairness of the American legal system. He fully believed that American justice would never allow his important work to be discontinued.

Whether from innocence or arrogance, or both, Reich severely underestimated the power of the FDA and its campaign against him. In February 1954 the FDA issued an injunction forbidding the interstate shipment of orgone accumulators. The injunction also denied the existence of orgone energy, and proclaimed that all Reich's books and publications were promotional material for the worthless accumulator.

As demanded by the terms of the injunction, Reich foolishly refused to appear in court. He was adamant that his scientific work could never be properly argued or evaluated in a law court. His legal counsel pleaded with Reich to reconsider, but he stood firm in his

position that he could not, in good conscience, defend his
life's work in court. His unyielding decision had
disastrous consequences.

The FDA won the injunction by default. The agency
was awarded the legal power to proceed with the
destruction of Reich's accumulators and all his published
writings.

The legal maneuverings culminated in a trial that
took place in Portland, Maine, in May 1956. Reich was
arrested in Washington, DC, on contempt of court
charges, and was forcibly brought to Portland in chains.
His refusal to cooperate with the courts over the
previous two years did not bode well with the judge.
However, Reich remained confident that higher authorities in the U.S. government would come to his rescue
and avert the impending court travesty.

Time was running out for Reich. Years earlier he had
been abandoned by Freud and the psychoanalytic
establishment. The communists drummed him out of the
Party, and the Nazis wanted him dead. He had offended
the Austrians, the Danes, the Swedes, and the Norwegians. Now the Americans would have their opportunity to
destroy the mad psychiatrist and his new god of orgone.

Reich was finally done in by the forces of the scientific
inquisition that rallied against him. He had played into
the hands of his enemies, and now they had him where
they wanted him. Reich was sentenced to two years in
federal prison.

Before imprisonment, the FDA had its final vengeance.
On June 5, 1956, the FDA officials came to Orgonon.
Reich and his young son Peter watched in silence as the
federal officials axed the accumulators. On June 26th,
Reich's books and journals at Orgonon were burned by
the government authorities. On August 23 in New York

City, the final destruction of Reich's literature took place. Six tons of books, journals, and papers were burned in a scientific holocaust. And not a single major newspaper in the Land of the Free protested this unprecedented action, so reminiscent of Nazi Germany.

In early March 1957, Reich was imprisoned at Danbury Federal Prison. The psychiatrist who examined Reich recorded his diagnosis, "Paranoia manifested by delusions of grandiosity and persecution and ideas of reference."[2] A few weeks later, Reich was transferred to the federal penitentiary at Lewisburg, Pennsylvania.

The United States government had won. Officially, orgone energy did not exist. Reich was certified as a mentally ill, quack psychiatrist who tried to foist a sex box and a cancer cure on the American public. The Reich affair was terminated.

One can only imagine the torment and loneliness that overtook Reich in his prison cell. Toward the end of October, Reich began to feel poorly, but he was afraid to bring the matter to the attention of the prison officials. He told friends that his jailers would try to kill him in prison, and he believed he would never get out of prison alive. On November 3, 1957, Reich was found dead in his cell, an apparent victim of a heart attack.

The body was taken to Orgonon for burial. A small band of loyal followers, including Ilse, Eva, and Peter, paid their last respects. Elsworth Baker MD, who had studied with Reich for eleven years, gave the eulogy.

"Friends, we are here to say farewell, a last farewell to Wilhelm Reich. Once in a thousand years, nay once in two thousand years, such a man comes upon this earth to change the destiny of the human race. As with all great men, distortion, falsehood, and persecution followed him. He met them all until an organized conspiracy sent him to prison and there killed him."[3]

Years later, Ellsworth Baker wrote, "Reich's attitude, in fact his entire life, was unconventional and as difficult for the world to understand as were his discoveries. Many legends, probably even religions, will develop about him. Already, some people look upon him as a superman who could not err, or a spaceman come to earth; others have rationalized and written articles attempting to prove him insane, a charlaton, or a fraud. Reich was not a mysterious superman nor a spaceman, nor was he insane or a fraud. He was very human, natural, and open, and foremost, a great and genuine scientist. He could be as soft and warm as a summer breeze or as violent and angry as a thunderstorm."[3]

It took me a long time to comprehend Reich and his achievements. I slowly realized that he alone had understood the full meaning and the significance of the cancer microbe. Long before Virginia and Eleanor, Reich had seen the tiny bacteria in cancer. He had gone far past my two friends by discovering the force that propelled these microbes to life. He was a visionary who perceived the energy that connected life to death — and death to life.

Was he a genius or a madman? There were few people who knew enough about the scope of his work to judge. Perhaps I was one of them. I had never experimented with hay grass infusions and protozoa, nor had I ever peered into microscopes that could magnify higher than 1000 times. But, like Reich, I had seen the cancer microbe and it had transformed my life. And so I admire and trust Reich the scientist.

For those who consider Reich an enemy of the people,

his official sins are duly recorded in the dusty archives of government office buildings in Vienna, Berlin, Copenhagen, Oslo and Washington.

For those who are willing to take the time to investigate Reich's work, a different sort of man emerges. It is my feeling that Reich desperately wanted to show the world that God existed in the realm of the orgone. Through the study of orgonomy, Reich believed man and science could prove, beyond doubt, that God is real. Like God, the orgone is indestructible. And like God, orgone energy exists everywhere in the universe. Man's spirit constantly reflects the orgone, eternally embued with new life rising from the ashes of death.

In some ways Reich was childlike and surprisingly naive. His downfall was overestimating the goodness of science; and underestimating the dark side of science. In human terms, he paid for this error with his life.

Of course, there are many who deny the dark forces of orthodox medical science. But they exist.

Of this I am sure. Because when I began to study the origin of AIDS, I encountered them.

References:

1. **Boadella D**: *Wilhelm Reich: The Evolution of His Work*. Vision Press, Chicago, 1973.

2. **Sharaf MR**: *Fury on Earth: A Biography of Wilhelm Reich*. St. Martin's Press/Marek, New York, 1983.

3. **Baker EF**: My eleven years with Reich. Journal of Orgonomy 18; 155-171, 1984.

CHAPTER THIRTEEN

AIDS and Biological Warfare

In 1979, the first case of a deadly new disease appeared in Manhattan, New York City. By 1981 several dozen additional cases were recorded. All the patients were young white gay men who had been previously healthy. The doctors were puzzled and their medications were useless against the onslaught of this rapidly fatal illness. Physicians had never witnessed such a devastating sickness that had a peculiar affinity for young homosexuals.

All the patients had severely damaged immune systems and no protection against microbes which produced life-threatening "opportunistic" infections. Purple cancerous tumors of Kaposi's sarcoma (KS) appeared on the skin of some of the men. KS is a rare form of cancer and most doctors had never seen a case. Suddenly, KS was appearing as a deadly marker in gays with this strange new disease.

Most of the men died of an opportunistic lung infection caused by a fungus known as Pneumocystis carinii. The fungal pneumonia became known as "gay" pneumonia; and KS as "gay cancer." Initially, the new disease was termed "gay-related immune deficiency" or GRID, for short. Privately, doctors were calling it the "gay plague."

The epidemic of AIDS (acquired immune deficiency syndrome) became official in 1981. Pneumocystis pneumonia and KS were designated as the two hallmark diseases required for a diagnosis of AIDS in "high risk" homosexual men. Government scientists began searching for a new "agent" to explain this new mystery disease. High on the list of suspects was a new virus, particularly one that could be transmitted sexually.

I had already found bacteria in KS tumors and I suspected that the cancer microbe was the mysterious "agent" in AIDS and "gay cancer." Before the epidemic, KS was an uncommon cancer discovered in Vienna in 1868 by the famous dermatologist, Moriz Kaposi. Before AIDS, KS was rarely fatal. However, during the 1950s KS was recognized as a common and more serious form of cancer in blacks in Central Africa. African KS is frequently fatal and the KS tumors often develop inside the body, as well as on the skin.

During the late 1970s I studied the skin tumors of three elderly heterosexual men with "classic" (pre-AIDS) KS. Cancer microbes were identified in acid-fast stained tissue sections of these tumors; and with the help of Dan Kelso, bacteria were cultured. Cancer bacteria were also discovered in the internal organs of an elderly white Los Angeles man who died from KS in 1973. Two papers on this KS research were published in 1981, the year AIDS became official [1,2]

When the epidemic broke out, U.S. government AIDS scientists theorized the new disease had its origin in central Africa because AIDS cases were uncovered there in the late 1970s. These African cases were indistinguishable from American AIDS cases in gays. Another "connection" was the similarity of "gay cancer" to the severe form of KS seen in African blacks.

In the early 1980s, AIDS cases were also discovered in Port-au-Prince, Haiti. The government AIDS experts theorized the AIDS agent was brought to Haiti from Central Africa. The disease was also supposedly brought to Manhattan by gay tourists who had sex with Haitian men. By 1983, most Americans blindly accepted the theory that American AIDS came from Africa. Eventually, the government theories became unalterable "facts."

Virginia Livingston had always said that cancer was infectious, but not contagious. I wondered if the microbe in KS had somehow mutated to become sexually transmissible. I examined the KS tumors and the enlarged lymph nodes of gays with AIDS. I also examined the autopsy tissue of homosexual men who died of this new syndrome. The cancer microbe was always present in the damaged tissues of these patients. In 1983, three more papers on cancer microbes in AIDS were published in reputable medical journals[3-5].

I thought surely the AIDS experts would pay attention to cancer bacteria that were so easy to detect in the AIDS-affected tissue. But my published research was ignored and never cited by the AIDS experts. By 1983 the government scientists were searching for a new virus, not for bacteria. The idea of a bacterial agent as the cause of AIDS was never considered. The cancer virologists were placed in charge of finding the cause of AIDS; and in the minds of the cancer virologists the cancer microbe did not exist.

In 1984, Robert Gallo of the National Cancer Institute announced that he had discovered the new virus that causes AIDS. The AIDS experts then proceeded to educate the doctors and the public about the new AIDS virus and its transmissibility.

The AIDS virus lives in the blood and the body fluids. The virus is a sexually transmitted retrovirus. In the form of an RNA virus, the AIDS retrovirus enters and infects a human cell. Once inside the cell, the virus has an enzyme (reverse transcriptase) that tranforms the RNA retrovirus into a DNA virus. The DNA form of the AIDS virus hides safely inside the normal DNA genetic material of the cell. When the "conditions" are appropriate, the dormant virus awakens and transforms itself back into the deadly RNA retrovirus form.

The virus in its activated RNA state multiplies wildly within the cell and kills it. Once set free from the cell the retrovirus enters another cell, and the killing process continues. The immune system is powerless against this clever virus. Once infected, the human body is infected forever. Although virologists never state it, the virus is "pleomorphic." It exists in one form outside the cell; and in another form inside the cell. It has only one function: to kill.

The AIDS retrovirus was initially called "human T-cell leukemia/lymphoma virus. The name was quickly changed to "human T-cell lymphotropic virus." Apparently the virologists did not want the public to connect the AIDS virus with well-known forms of cancer, such as leukemia and lymphoma. Although the AIDS virus is definitely a cancer-causing virus, the AIDS scientists have stressed that AIDS is not cancer. This scientific double-talk is further intended to make the public believe that AIDS is a disease totally unrelated to cancer.

The AIDS virus can be transmitted from person-to-person by sex and by blood and blood products. A blood test has been devised to screen-out infected AIDS blood. Consequently, blood transfusion is relatively safe, unless a donor is "incubating" the virus and reacts as "negative" to the AIDS blood test. Prior to the screening of AIDS-infected blood, many hemophiliacs became infected with the virus. Similarly, other people have also acquired the virus through contaminated blood transfusions. Needle-sharing intravenous drug abusers are highly susceptible to AIDS. And an infected pregnant woman can pass the virus on to her unborn child.

After laboring for one year to precisely "classify" the AIDS virus, a scientific committee gave the virus a new name in 1986. The reclassified AIDS virus is now officially known as "human immunodeficiency virus" or HIV, for short.

By the late 1980s most nations were reporting AIDS cases. The epidemic that started in the late 1970s in New York City, Central Africa and Haiti, is no longer a gay or a black disease, or a disease of hemophiliacs or drug addicts. The AIDS virus is everywhere. . . and no one is immune.

Where did the AIDS virus come from? The "introduction" of the AIDS virus onto the planet is unprecedented. The cancer virologists and the government epidemiologists have declared that the virus originated in the African green monkey. The monkey virus purportedly had "jumped species" and entered the black population. From there it migrated to Haiti and Manhattan.

African AIDS primarily affects heterosexuals. After the virus "entered the black population" it spread to millions of blacks because of blood transfusions, dirty needles, promiscuity and "genital ulcers" — or so they said.

Not everyone believes the official government story, although it is rare to find people who express this view publicly. A popular underground theory is that AIDS is biological warfare: AIDS has nothing to do with green monkeys or homosexuality or drug addiction or genital ulcerations or anal sex or promiscuity. It has to do with scientists experimenting on blacks and gays. And it is covered-up genocide.

The scientific community regards the AIDS biowarfare theory as paranoid thinking and as communist-inspired disinformation. I thought that way too, until I met Robert Strecker MD in the summer of 1986.

Virginia Livingston introduced me to Bob Strecker. She heard he was spreading the accusation that AIDS was biowarfare. She wanted to know more about his ideas, and invited me to her home to meet him.

Strecker believes AIDS has nothing to do with green monkeys. On the contrary, he is convinced the AIDS virus was genetically engineered in a high-tech cancer virus lab. The appearance, structure, and molecular weight of the virus indicate the AIDS virus is a genetic recombinant of two viruses spliced together to create a deadly hybrid virus designed to destroy the immune system. In Strecker's view, the AIDS virus most closely resembles two well-known viruses: bovine leukemia virus of cattle, and visna virus of sheep. Visna causes brain rot in sheep.

Strecker claims the "introduction" of the AIDS virus into millions of African blacks correlates with smallpox vaccination programs sponsored by the World Health Organization (the WHO). During the years 1966-1977, the WHO launched a global smallpox eradication program that resulted in the administration of 24,000 million (2.4 billion) doses of smallpox vaccine. The smallpox vaccine is prepared from cows experimentally infected with vaccinia (cowpox) virus. Strecker insists the smallpox vaccines were accidentally (or deliberately) contaminated with an AIDS-causing virus which produced the African AIDS holocaust.

What about gays in America? Why were Manhattan

gays the first to get AIDS? Strecker's answer is simple: the gays got the AIDS virus through the hepatitis B experimental vaccine program sponsored by the government.

What about the AIDS "connection" to Africa? "There isn't any, " Strecker said. "It's all a big cover-up to hide the real truth."

I was dumbfounded. Strecker continued. "If you carefully study the roots of AIDS, the biowarfare theory is the only one that makes any sense. But be careful! What you read will surprise and shock the hell out of you. You will read about military biowarfare experiments, and animal cancer experiments that will sicken your stomach. And when you finish all this — you will know what I say is true."

My year-long investigation of Strecker's theory resulted in the 1988 publication of *AIDS AND THE DOCTORS OF DEATH: AN INQUIRY INTO THE ORIGIN OF THE AIDS EPIDEMIC*[6]. The investigation also shattered many of my illusions about cancer research, animal virus experimentation, and the new genetic engineering biotechnology. It was a personal rite of passage that forever etched my soul with the madness of high tech biomedical science.

Was AIDS biowarfare? What I learned about secret human experimentation and biowarfare chilled me to the marrow.

In 1932 a medical experiment, conducted by the U.S Public Health Service, was undertaken on four hundred poor, illiterate black sharecroppers in Tuskegee, Alabama. All the men had syphilis. The doctors who carried out the experiment lied to the men and their families, telling them only that they were suffering from "bad blood." Under the watchful eye of the government and the medical establishment, the Tuskegee experiment lasted 40 years.

The racist experiment was as simple as it was diabolic. The physicians wanted to know what would happen to the health of these men if treatment for syphilis was withheld. The doctors assured the men they would look after their "bad blood" and provide for all their health care, free of charge.

When a penicillin cure for syphilis became available in the 1940s, the men were not treated because treatment would ruin the medical experiment. Throughout their lives the men never knew they had a serious, life-threatening venereal disease. Some of the men sexually transmitted syphilis to their wives and lovers. Some of the babies born of these infected women were syphilitic. When each man died, the experimenters offered money for funeral and burial expenses with the proviso that the family permit an autopsy at the special hospital involved in the study.

During the Black Civil Rights Movement of the 1960s, intense political pressure was put on the government to stop this unethical, racist experiment. In 1972 the syphilis study was finally terminated. The definitive account of the Tuskegee syphilis study appears in *BAD BLOOD*, by James H. Jones[7]. Martin P. Levine has also written about this shocking study with genocidal overtones ("Bad blood," *New York Native*, February 16, 1987). Levine emphasizes that the Tuskegee experiment was supervised by the Centers for Disease Control (CDC), the same government agency that now oversees the AIDS epidemic.

In Manchuria in the late 1930s and early 1940s, the

Japanese performed the most diabolic biological experiments ever performed on human beings. When the Japanese overran the country, they established a biowarfare research and production facility in Pingfan, near the city of Harbin. General Shiro Ishii was placed in charge of the infamous biowarfare installation.

According to Charles Pillar and Keith Yamamoto (*GENE WARS: MILITARY CONTROL OVER THE NEW GENETIC TECHNOLOGIES*), "At least 3000 Chinese, Korean, Soviet, American, British, and Austalian prisoners of war died horrific deaths at the hands of the Pingfan technicians." In the biowarfare experiments the Japanese deliberately infected prisoners with microbes causing cholera, dysentery, typhoid, syphilis and other infectious diseases. "The work included trials of anthrax and gas gangrene bombs. Prisoners were tied to stakes, their buttocks exposed to the shrapnel flying from a bomb detonated by remote control. The course of the disease was meticulously tracked and recorded as the victims died in agony. Other prisoners were infected with organisms causing cholera and plague, only to be dissected — sometimes while still alive — to monitor the progressive degeneration of their internal organs."[8]

To this day the Japanese deny these biowarfare atrocities, as well as countless others performed in China during World War Two. A slight hint of these Japanese war crimes against China appears in the 1988 Oscar-winning film, THE LAST EMPEROR. The "offending" footage in the film was removed for screenings in Japan.

During the Japanese war crime trials the American military learned the full details of General Ishii's death experiments. However, the Army feared the Russians might benefit from learning about the Japanese biowarfare experiments. To thwart this possibility, the U.S.

Army made a deal: If Ishii willingly turned over his data to the Army biowarfare department, the U.S. government would not prosecute him, nor would they turn him over to the Russians. Ishii agreed. The biowarfare case against the Japanese was dropped.

Further details of this gross miscarriage of justice are recorded in *A HIGHER FORM OF KILLING* (1982). According to Robert Harris and Jeremy Paxman's book, "The Americans were clearly stunned by the (biological warfare) information. The experiments were as horrific as any conducted by the Nazis, yet the Camp Detrick (Maryland) specialists dispassionately concluded in their summary of the report of Biowarfare Investigations of 12 December 1947 that the potential benefits of the research for Western biological warfare program far outweighed the demands of justice. If the Japanese were to be questioned by the Russians, then they rather than the Americans would obtain the benefits of wartime research. This concern to spare the Japanese doctors possible 'embarassment' found a ready response in Washington, where, in order to maintain a lead over Soviet plans for germ warfare, the full extent of American knowledge of Japanese wartime plans was kept secret for thirty years."[9]

In the 1950s and 60s the Army and the CIA conducted secret experiments against U.S civilian and military personnel. In recent years the sordid details of these experiments (some of which ended in murder) have come to light.

Today, all the major powers in the world experiment with covert biological warfare. Only a fool would believe otherwise.

In 1969 a riot erupted when police attempted to unfairly

arrest homosexuals outside a gay bar called Stonewall in the Greenwich Village section of Manhattan. Scores of gays and lesbians gathered on the Village streets to protest the arrests, and the riots took several days to quell. The Stonewall experience contributed to the birth of the gay liberation movement of the 1970s. The aim of the movement was to secure full protection of civil rights and liberties for homosexuals.

During the 1970s many gays came out of the closet, and Gay Pride parades in New York, San Francisco and Los Angeles became annual events. Tens of thousands of happy and normal-looking homosexuals appeared on television screens throughout America. Not everyone was pleased. Many heterosexuals were convinced they were witnessing the resurrection of Sodom and Gomorrah.

In the same year as the Stonewall riots, a spokesman for the Department of Defense told a Congressional Hearing that a "super germ" could be developed as part of our experimental biowarfare program. This genetically engineered germ would be very different from any previous microbe known to mankind. The agent would be a highly effective killing agent because the immune system would be powerless against this supermicrobe. (Testimony before a "Subcommittee of the Committee on Appropriations, House of Representatives, Department of Defense Appropriations for 1970, dated July 1, 1969, Washington).

A transcript of this meeting on "Synthetic Biological Agents" reads as follows: "There are two things about the biological agent field I would like to mention. One is the possibility of technological surprise. Molecular biology is a field that is advancing rapidly, and eminent biologists believe that WITHIN A PERIOD OF 5 TO

10 YEARS IT WOULD BE POSSIBLE TO PRODUCE A SYNTHETIC BIOLOGICAL AGENT, AN AGENT THAT DOES NOT NATURALLY EXIST AND FOR WHICH NO NATURAL IMMUNITY COULD HAVE BEEN ACQUIRED. (Author's italics.)

Mr. Sikes. Are we doing any work in that field?

Dr. MacArthur. We are not.

Mr. Sikes. Why not? Lack of money or lack of interest?

Dr. MacArthur. CERTAINLY NOT LACK OF INTEREST.

Mr. Sikes. Would you provide for our records information on what would be required, what the advantages of such a program would be, the time and cost involved?

Dr. MacArthur. We will be happy to.

(The information follows:)

"THE DRAMATIC PROGRESS BEING MADE IN THE FIELD OF MOLECULAR BIOLOGY LED US TO INVESTIGATE THE RELEVANCE OF THIS FIELD OF SCIENCE TO BIOLOGICAL WARFARE. A small group of experts considered this matter and provided the the following observations:

1. All biological agents up to the present time are representatives of naturally occurring disease, and are thus known by scientists throughout the world. They are easily available to qualified scientists for research, EITHER FOR OFFENSIVE OR DEFENSIVE PURPOSES.

2. WITHIN THE NEXT 5 TO 10 YEARS, IT WOULD PROBABLY BE POSSIBLE TO MAKE A NEW INFECTIVE MICROORGANISM WHICH COULD DIFFER IN CERTAIN IMPORTANT ASPECTS FROM ANY KNOWN DISEASE-CAUSING

ORGANISMS. MOST IMPORTANT OF THESE IS THAT IT MIGHT BE REFRACTORY TO THE IMMUNOLOGICAL AND THERAPEUTIC PROCESSES UPON WHICH WE DEPEND TO MAINTAIN OUR RELATIVE FREEDOM FROM INFECTIOUS DISEASE.

3. A research program to explore the feasibility of this could be completed in approximately 5 years at a total cost of $10 million.

4. It would be very difficult to establish such a program. Molecular biology is a relatively new science. There are not many competent scientists in the field, almost all are in UNIVERSITY LABORATORIES, and they are generally adaquately supported form sources other than the Department of Defense. However, it was considered possible to initiate an adequate program through THE NATIONAL ACADEMY OF SCIENCES—NATIONAL RESEARCH COUNCIL (NAS-NRC).

The matter was discussed with the NAS-NRC, and TENTATIVE PLANS WERE MADE TO INITIATE THE PROGRAM. However, decreasing finds in CB (chemical/biological), growing criticism of the CB program, and our reluctance to involve the NAS-NRC in such a controversial endeavor have led us to postpone it for the past 2 years.

IT IS A HIGHLY CONTROVERSIAL ISSUE AND THERE ARE MANY WHO BELIEVE SUCH RESEARCH SHOULD NOT BE UNDERTAKEN LEST IT LEAD TO YET ANOTHER METHOD OF MASSIVE KILLING OF LARGE POPULATIONS. On the other hand, without the sure scientific knowledge that such a weapon is possible, and an understanding of the ways it could be done, there is little that can be done to devise defensive measures. Should an enemy develop it there is little doubt that this is an important area of potential military technological inferiority in which there is no adequate research program."

During the late 1960s, the U.S. Army's biological warfare program intensified, particularly in the area of DNA and "gene splicing" research. In order to placate the fears of critics, President Richard Nixon renounced germ warfare, except for "medical defensive research."

In 1971 Nixon ordered that a major part of the Army's Biological Warfare Unit be transferred over to the National Cancer Institute (NCI). In 1971 Nixon also initiated his famous War on Cancer. Utilizing the latest techniques of genetic engineering and laboratory cell culture, the cancer virologists learned how to "jump" animal cancer viruses from one species of animal into another. Chicken viruses were put into lamb kidney cells. Baboon viruses were spliced into human blood cells. The combinations were endless. In the process, new forms of cancer, immunodeficiency, and opportunistic infections were produced in the animals.

As predicted by the biowarfare experts, new cancer-causing monster viruses were created that had a deadly affect on the immune system. In one government-sponsored experiment reported in 1974, newborn chimpanzees were taken away from their mothers at birth and weaned on milk obtained from virus-infected cows. Some of the chimps sickened and died with two new diseases that had never been observed in chimpanzees. The first was a fungal pneumonia known as *Pneumocystis carinii* pneumonia (the "gay pneumonia" of AIDS); the second was leukemia [10].

Dr. Strecker believes that some cancer virologists were not adverse to experimenting secretly with humans, particularly African blacks. To substantiate this claim, he referred me to a 1972 "Committee Report" in the Federation Proceedings [11]. The report was based on a July 1970 workshop sponsored by the National Institutes of Health and the WHO. In order to apply experimental cancer virus research to humans, the Committee "visualized" several "useful experimental approaches" for studying the human immune system. The scientists suggested that people could be injected "with well-defined bacterial and viral antigens during preventative vaccinations. This approach would be particularly informative when applied to sibships."

In simple English, the word "sibships" refers to children of the same family. "During preventative vaccination" most certainly means that children and adults would be given experimental infectious agents (i.e. "bacterial and viral antigens") along with routine (i.e. "preventative") vaccinations. The human population for experimentation was not stated. However, poor African blacks are often used as research subjects for international health agencies. Such programs offer alleged health benefits for third world children. Over 400,000 third world children die yearly of malnutrition, diarrhea, and infectious disease. In the event of an experimental vaccine mishap, it is not likely that the parents of third-world children would seek legal recourse.

A few scientists expressed concern regarding the safety of laboratories housing these dangerous mutant viruses and supergerms. What would happen if one of these deadly, genetically engineered microbes escaped from the laboratory?

In November 1973 a high-level conference entitled "Biohazards in Biological Research" convened at Asilomar, near Pacific Grove in Northern California. The leading cancer virologists freely admitted there was no foolproof way to prevent the escape of these cancer-causing viruses into the community. However, in the event of an "accident," plans were drawn up to insure that the "introduction" of such a virus into the human population could be detected and investigated.

At the conference, sophisticated epidemiologic studies were devised. Government agencies would oversee groups or "cohorts" of people "who might be exposed in the future" or "who had been previously exposed" to the cancer-causing virus. The researchers at Asilomar were well aware of the grave risks of their cancer virus research. However, they also understood that their mission was to prove, beyond all doubt, that these animal viruses caused cancer in humans.

Scientists like Francis Black of Yale University Medical School were not averse to taking risks. "If we do believe in our mission of trying to control cancer, it behooves us to accept some risk. Even if, as has been suggested, five or ten people might lose their lives, this might be a small price for the number of lives that would be saved[12]." Science and Ethics had "officially" now parted company.

By the mid-1970s the government scientists were taking a keen interest in the health of gay men. The government epidemiologists quickly provided the statistical data to "prove" that gays were promiscuous and that VD was rampant in the homosexual community. (In retrospect, the health of the gay community in the 1970s was excellent when compared to the tens of thousands of AIDS deaths in gays in the 1980s.) A decade later, in 1989, the sexually-transmitted disease experts estimated there were 1-2 million cases of gonorrhea annually; 4 million cases of chlamydia; 12 million human wart papilloma virus cases; and 20 to 30 million cases of genital herpes. Most of these sexually transmitted disease cases are heterosexual.

In the early 1970s, researchers learned that the virus causing hepatitis B could be spread sexually. Not surprisingly, epidemiologists discovered a high rate of hepatitis B infection in gay men. An experimental vaccine against hepatitis B was developed and tested in chimpanzees. When it was ready for human testing, the epidemiologists decided that young gay promiscuous men would be the ideal "cohort" to test the vaccine's efficacy.

Wolf Szmuness, a Polish physician trained in the Soviet Union, was placed in charge of the hepatitis B vaccine program. Under peculiar circumstances, Szmuness defected to the U.S. in 1969[6]. He arrived penniless and jobless, and with a poor knowledge of the English language. He was hired on at a low paying position at the New York City Blood Center in Manhattan. Within five years he became head of the Laboratory of Epidemiology at the Center, and was awarded millions of dollars in government grants to support his hepatitis research. He was also appointed Professor of Epidemiology at Columbia University. In the late 1970s a bloodmobile began canvassing the gay ghetto in Greenwich Village, looking for homosexual volunteers for Szmuness' experiment. Over ten thousand Manhattan gays signed-up.

Szmuness was highly selective in the men he chose for the final experiment. The cohort had to be composed of young, responsible, healthy, intelligent, preferably white, promiscuous gays and bisexuals. The men had to have an address and a phone number, and be willing to provide blood samples over a long period of time. The hepatitis B experiment was a costly one. The Centers for Disease Control (CDC), the National Institutes of Health (NIH), and the National Institute of Allergy and Infectious Diseases were all involved in the study, as well as the big pharmaceutical money interests. Szmuness didn't want any uncooperative or hard-to-find gays screwing up his experiment. There was too much money at stake.

The gay experiment began in November 1978 at the New York City Blood Center in Manhattan. Over one thousand men took part in the vaccine study.

November 1978 was a cataclysmic month. In early November, astrologers were perplexed by the highly unusual configuration of seven heavenly bodies in the secretive sign of Scorpio. The Sun and the Moon, and Saturn, Mars, Venus, Mercury, and Uranus, were all housed in Scorpio — the sign of sex, death, and transformation.

At the beginning of the month, Reverend Jim Jones commanded his thousand American followers to drink poison as an act of protest. The mass suicide in Jonestown, Guyana, stunned the world. In late November at City Hall, Harvey Milk (an avowed homosexual and an elected city supervisor) and George Moscone (the heterosexual Mayor of San Francisco) were gunned down in cold blood by a political assassin who hated gays.

In January 1979, a few months after Wolf Szmuness began his hepatitis experiment in Manhattan, a young white gay man in the Village became seriously ill. Purple lesions of KS appeared on his body and he died horribly. During the next thirty months, Manhattan doctors uncovered dozens more cases. All the men were young and white and gay. A decade later, AIDS became the leading cause of death in young men and women in New York City.

The secrets of Scorpio reveal themselves slowly, and only the most perceptive are privy to the hidden knowledge of sex and death that is contained within the most occult sign of the zodiac. AIDS in America began under the influence of this powerful planetary stellium in Scorpio. In November 1978 only the mystics could have foretold the evil forces that would seek to destroy sex on the planet. However, if one carefully studies the fate of the gays who were drawn into Wolf Szmuness' experiment, it is obvious that AIDS was unleashed in Manhattan during that fateful month.

Wolf Szmuness was thrilled with the success of his hepatitis B experiment. In March 1980 the CDC sponsored additional experiments involving gays in San Francisco, Los Angeles, Denver, St. Louis, and Chicago. In the fall of 1980 the first case of AIDS appeared in a young gay man living in San Francisco.

Six months later, in June 1981, the AIDS epidemic became "official." Physicians could not understand why young, white, previously healthy homosexual men were dying mysteriously in Manhattan, San Francisco, and Los Angeles.

In December 1981, the CDC sent a team of epidemiologists to Denmark to study Danish gays who had sex with Manhattan gays during the period 1980-1981[13]. In 1982 the CDC covertly tested the blood of male patients in the medical offices of Manhattan and Washington D.C. physicians, whose clientele was "90% likely to be gay or bisexual." The researchers suspected that Washington gays who had sex with New York men might be "immune deficient." This study, published in 1985, proved that the CDC's hypothesis was correct[14]. These early 1981-1982 epidemiologic studies suggest that U.S. government scientists were well-aware of the extreme communicability of the new mystery agent that was "introduced" into the gay community.

A few months after his discovery of the AIDS virus, Robert Gallo of the National Cancer Institute was interviewed by James D'Eramo in the *New York Native* (September 9, 1984). D'Eramo asked Gallo to explain why AIDS primarily targeted gay men. Gallo retorted that the same question might be asked about Legionnaire's disease, which attacked conventioners housed in a Philadelphia hotel in 1976. (The cause was finally proven to be bacteria blown into the hotel rooms by bacteria-contaminated water in the air-conditioning system.) Gallo reasoned: "Why were they Legionnaires? They were Legionnaires because they were the ones exposed." He continued his logic in finally answering D'Eramo's original question. "They are homosexuals because they were the ones exposed. Forget all the other hocus-pocus. They are the people who were exposed. Why them? No one knows. . . It was acquired. You can make a best guess. What would your guess be? Mine would be only what I read in the newspapers."

Gallo was quite sure the AIDS virus came from Africa. "Many organisms and viruses had their origins in Africa. There's a great zoology in Africa, isn't there?"

D'Eramo asked Gallo how he regarded my reports of bacteria in KS. Gallo evaded any direct comment on my cancer microbe research, and simply responded, "I don't know the cause of KS."

D'Eramo continued. "Why does AIDS-related KS occur in gay men?" The world's leading AIDS experts answered, "I don't know. KS confuses me."

What about sex? "I would advise sexual abstinence until this problem is solved. It may be a while. It may be a lifetime. I'm sorry. I'm doing my best."

Shortly after Gallo declared himself the discoverer of the AIDS virus in April 1984, Luc Montagnier insisted he had discovered the AIDS virus a year before Gallo. In January 1983 Montagnier, a researcher at the Pasteur Institute in Paris, sent an AIDS virus to Gallo's lab for identification. Montagnier's virus was isolated from the swollen lymph nodes of a gay Parisian who had had sex in Manhattan in 1979.

Montagnier and the Pasteur Institute accused Gallo of stealing the French virus and presenting it to the academic world as his own. The French declared that they deserved to be recognized as the true discoverers of the AIDS virus. Gallo denied the charge, insisting that Montagnier's virus was not the true AIDS virus. The CDC concurred by emphasizing that the French virus and Gallo's AIDS virus were two completely different viruses. Eventually, the two "different" viruses were proven to be identical.

The top American scientists repeatedly theorized that AIDS originated in Africa: the AIDS virus had been in Africa for years, and maybe for centuries. As proof of this, the AIDS experts said that old 1950s African blood specimens tested positive for the virus. Later, these reports proved erroneous when other investigators could not confirm the blood findings. Furthermore, physicians in Africa insisted there were no cases of proven AIDS until the late 1970s, around the same time that cases were diagnosed in Manhattan gays.

In 1988 Montagnier noted that "there is no evidence of any reservoir of species of monkey that is truly positive for HIV (the AIDS virus)." Admitting that the origin of the AIDS virus is "a continuing mystery," he added, "Some very weak arguments are used to place the origin of HIV in Africa. One is the discovery of AIDS virus in serum samples taken from a woman in Zaire before 1970, but that isn't so long ago, and does not prove the virus first sprang from that region. We have to be very careful in assessing the origin of this virus, which is really mysterious" (*Skin and Allergy News*, January 1988).

In spite of all this, Robert Gallo and Myron Essex (a Harvard veterinarian whose expertise is animal cancer experimentation) continue to promote the idea that AIDS originated in Africa. Their idea has been disproven by a 1986 study of elderly Ugandans who were "sexually inactive for the past five years." When tested for AIDS virus antibodies, none of the old people in Uganda's largest city were positive![15]. In addition, when the blood of African KS patients was tested, most patients had no evidence of AIDS virus infection! This indicates that KS in Africa is not directly related to AIDS virus infection. Furthermore, there is no "connection" between African KS and American AIDS, except in the minds of retrovirologists like Gallo and Essex. It has already been stated that Gallo was unable to distinguish between two identical AIDS viruses. In addition, both Essex and Gallo have erred by proclaiming the "discovery" of new "human" AIDS-like viruses that were later proven to be old "contaminant animal viruses" originating from their own laboratories.

Angry Africans accuse white "racist" scientists of trying to blame blacks for starting AIDS; and some black leaders insist the African origin of AIDS is a lie concocted by American scientists to cover-up the fact that AIDS is biowarfare against Africans.

In 1985 the Pasteur Institute filed suit against the U.S. Federal Government. The French argued that they were the true discoverers of the virus, and they wanted their full share of the profits to be derived from the new AIDS industry. The French lawyers hinted about scientific irregularities and alterations of scientific documents on the part of the Americans. The lawyers were also aware that Gallo had previously made serious errors in virus identification. Gallo's 1975 "discovery" of a "new" and "human" HL23 virus proved to be three different contaminating ape viruses (gibbon-ape virus, simian sarcoma virus, and baboon endogenous virus). Gallo claims he has no idea how these viruses could have contaminated his research on HL23.

Other legal evidence was even more damaging. Gallo had repeatedly stated that Montagnier's virus was not the real AIDS virus. However, further investigation proved the two viruses were as identical as any two viruses could be. The French lawyers could easily prove that Gallo stole Montagnier's AIDS virus.

In early 1987, the French Premier and President Ronald Reagan intervened in the increasingly delicate matter. Behind closed doors, it was conceded that debating AIDS science in court would open a big can of worms. Particularly delicate was the biowarfare issue. And neither government wanted any hint of biowarfare aired in public. A quick settlement was reached out of court for an undisclosed sum. The French were accepted as co-discovers of the AIDS virus. And the public missed the scientific scandal of the century.

———

A decade after the epidemic began, most people still believe the "official" African green monkey story. Inconsistent with this theory is the fact that AIDS cases were initially discovered in Africa, Haiti, and in Manhattan during the same time period in the late 1970s.

The AIDS medical establishment unquestioningly accepts the notion that a black African heterosexual AIDS epidemic transformed itself into a young white male homosexual epidemic in Manhattan. How is this biologically possible? In truth, the transformation of a black heterosexual epidemic into an exclusively white American homosexual epidemic is not biologically possible. Nevertheless, the leading AIDS experts carefully avoid all discussion of this issue. They claim the exact origin of AIDS is irrelevant: the important issue is finding a cure for the disease.

A few cracks in the monkey theory have appeared in print. A news story entitled "Research refutes idea that human AIDS virus originated in monkey" appeared in the *Los Angeles Times* (June 2, 1988). In the process of decoding the genetic structure of the monkey virus and the human AIDS virus, Japanese molecular biologists discovered that the gene sequences of the two viruses differed by more than 50%. This indicates absolutely no genetic relationship between the green monkey and the AIDS virus. The scientific conclusion of the Japanese was completely at odds with the official U.S. story proclaimed by the two leading AIDS experts, Gallo and Essex. The Japanese investigators specifically criticized Myron Essex and Phyllis Kanki of Harvard Medical School, who "discovered" a second AIDS virus in African green monkeys that was widely heralded in medical circles and in the media. Essex and Kanki's "second" AIDS virus was later proven to be another "contaminant" virus. The origin of the contaminant monkey virus was traced to the Harvard researchers own laboratory.

If the human AIDS virus is not related to the African green monkey virus, what is its origin? According to *The Los Angeles Times* medical writer, Robert Steinbrook, "the new (Japanese) findings lend support to other explanations for the origins of human AIDS viruses. These include their beginnings in common ancestors of humans and primates, their presence in isolated human populations for hundreds or thousands of years, or the existence of a yet-to-be identified prototype AIDS-like virus that first infected humans in modern times." I tried to understand what the newswriter meant by this, but it sounded like double-talk to cover-up fuzzy scientific thinking and the real truth about AIDS.

On November 13, 1988, *The Orange County Register* devoted an entire section of the newspaper to AIDS in Africa. Several African officials were interviewed. All were adamant that AIDS did not originate in Africa. The theory "is false and has never been scientifically proved, so why should Africa be the scapegoat?" declared Dr. Didace Nzaramba, director of the AIDS prevention program in Rwanda.

The Register commented: "From early on, scientists have speculated that the disease might have begun in

Africa. Researchers in Africa tested old blood samples and said they found HIV-infected serum that went back years. In 1985, Harvard researchers, Phyllis Kanki and Myron Essex, announced the discovery of a new virus isolated in green monkeys that seemed similar to HIV. Eventually, researchers concluded that early blood tests used in Africa were not totally reliable, and Kanki and Essex said their blood tests probably had been contaminated and that their results were invalid. But the perception of an African link was established."

Was the AIDS virus injected into American gays during Szmuness' hepatitis B vaccine experiment? And why did the U.S. government choose Wolf Szmuness, a Soviet-trained doctor and a recent American immigrant, to head this dangerous experiment? June Goodfield has written the definitive account of the gay hepatitis experiment in her book, *QUEST FOR THE KILLERS* (1985)[16]. According to Goodfield, Szmuness had a painful life. During World War Two, he was held as a political prisoner in Siberia, and was repeatedly interrogated and beaten by the Russian KGB for refusing to cooperate in spy activities. When he could not be broken, they warned him: "Say nothing of this to anyone, but remember. We will reach you anywhere in the world. No matter where you go, no matter where you go, no matter where you try to hide, you will never be out of our grasp."[16] The full story of Szmuness' strange life remains an enigma.

    Dr. Szmuness' experimental hepatitis B vaccine was manufactured by the National Institute of Health (NIH) and by the Merck drug company. During the clinical trial Szmuness was concerned about possible vaccine contamination. According to Goodfield, "This was no theoretical fear, contamination having been suspected in one vaccine batch made by the National Institutes of Health, though never in Merck's."[16] As previously mentioned, there are scientific connections between the NIH and the military biowarfare department. Furthermore, the Merck company is no stranger to biological warfare research. George Merck, who once headed the company, "led American research into germ weapons during the Second World War."[9]

Through the testing of blood specimens donated by the gay volunteers of the hepatitis B cohort, the government epidemiologists were able to detect the "introduction" and the spread of the AIDS virus in the gay community. Tens of thousands of blood samples drawn from thirteen thousand gay men are stored at the New York City Blood Center. Szmuness insisted that all these specimens be retained. When asked why he was keeping so many vials of blood, Szmuness replied, "Because one day another disease may erupt and we'll need this material"[16]. Within a few months AIDS cases appeared in Manhattan. Several years later when Szmuness' gay blood samples were tested for AIDS virus antibodies, it was discovered that the AIDS virus was "introduced" into the gay population of New York City sometime around 1978-1979, the exact year that Szmuness' experiment began. Did Szmuness have the psychic ability to accurately predict that a new disease would appear in the gay community, or did he know that the AIDS virus was being introduced into his volunteers? Unfortunately, the answers to these questions can only be surmised. In June 1982, Wolf Szmuness died of lung cancer.

Was AIDS introduced into millions of Africans during

government-sponsored smallpox vaccine programs?
Animal and human cells harbor all sorts of viruses,
including viruses not yet discovered. Animal tissue cell
cultures are often used in the manufacture of viral
vaccines. Therefore, the possibility of vaccine contamination with an animal virus is a constant danger in the
pharmaceutical production of vaccines.

Despite the most meticulous precautions in manufac-
turing human vaccines, contaminating animal viruses
are known to survive the vaccine process. For example,
during the 1950s millions of people were injected with
polio vaccines contaminated with "SV 40" — a cancer-
causing monkey virus. Such vaccine contamination
problems are kept hidden from the public. Yet in spite of
the known danger, drug companies and physicians pooh-
pooh any suggestion that AIDS could have arisen from
virus-contaminated vaccines.

Animal cancer viruses are also contained in fetal calf
serum, a serum commonly used as a laboratory nutrient
to feed animal and human tissue cell cultures. Viruses in
calf serum can be carried over as "contaminants" into
the final vaccine product.

The problem of vaccine contamination by fetal calf
serum and its relationship to AIDS is the subject of J.
Grote's letter ("Bovine visna virus and the origin of the
AIDS epidemic") published in the October 1988 *Journal
of the Royal (London) Society of Medicine*. Grote
discounts the green monkey theory and questions
whether "bovine visna virus" contamination of labora-
tory-used fetal bovine serum could cause AIDS. Bovine
visna virus is similar in appearance to the AIDS (HIV)
virus. Grote, a London-based AIDS researcher, writes:
"The seriousness of this becomes apparent when we
consider that the manufacture of vaccines requires the

growth of virus in cell cultures using fetal calf serum in the growth medium. The contamination of vaccines with adventitious viruses has been of concern for many years and the presence of virus-like structures in 'virus-screened' bovine serum has also been reported. It seems absolutely vital that all vaccines are screened for HIV prior to use and that bovine visna virus is further investigated as to its relationship to HIV and its possible causal role in progression towards AIDS."

Millions of African blacks are now infected with the AIDS virus. This large number could never have been infected by the simple act of a monkey virus "jumping" over to infect one African. The most logical explanation to account for the millions of Africans infected is that the vaccines used in the WHO mass inoculation programs were contaminated.

Was the contamination accidental or deliberate? It is well-known that the vaccinia (cowpox) virus used in the manufacture of the smallpox vaccine is an excellent virus for genetic engineering. For example. "researchers have been able to splice genes coding for the surface coats of other viruses, such as influenza, hepatitis, and rabies — into vaccinia virus DNA. The result: a 'broad spectrum' vaccine with a coat of many colors[8]. Regarding the Soviet claim that AIDS is a U.S. biowarfare experiment, Pillar and Yamamoto comment that "Although no evidence has been presented to support this claim, manipulating genes to defeat the body's immune response is quite feasible."[8]

During the years 1960-1977, the WHO administered 24,000 million doses of smallpox vaccine worldwide. Could any of these vaccine batches have been contaminated with a genetically engineered virus designed for biowarfare purposes? According to Allan Chase's

MAGIC SHOTS (1982)[17], "The Soviet Union donated 140 million doses; the United States 40 million doses; twenty other nations combined to donate another 220 million doses." The remaining two billion doses of smallpox vaccine were made in newly-established laboratories in third world countries, with the help of WHO specialists.

Since 1985, *The Executive Intelligence Review*, a publication of the now-imprisoned Lyndon LaRouche, has been claiming that the Soviets are involved in extensive research capable of producing the AIDS virus[18]. It is claimed that U.S. AIDS policy "is dictated by the Soviet government, through Soviet control over the infectious-disease bureaucracy of the WHO." *The Review* further states "The WHO Communicable Disease Division, which coordinates all AIDS and other lethal disease work internationally, is headed and manned by a Soviet nest of infectious disease specialists." While the Russians are accusing America of starting AIDS, LaRouche fears the communists are covertly carrying out their own biowarfare agenda.

On May 11, 1987, *The London Times*, one of the world's most respected newspapers, published an explosive article entitled, "Smallpox vaccine triggered AIDS virus." The story suggests that African AIDS is a direct outgrowth of the WHO smallpox eradication program. The smallpox vaccine allegedly awakened a "dormant" AIDS virus infection in the black population. According to Robert Gallo, "The link between the WHO program and the epidemic is an interesting and important hypothesis. I cannot say that it actually happened, but I have been saying for some years that the use of live vaccines such as that used for smallpox can activate a dormant infection such as HIV (the AIDS virus)." *The*

Times story is one of the most important stories ever printed on the AIDS epidemic; yet the story was killed and never appeared in any major U.S. newspaper.

Despite all the known information on biowarfare and secret human experimentation, as well as the genetic engineering of superviruses and the vaccine contamination problems, the medical establishment ignores all discussion of the AIDS biowarfare issue. In the prestigious *British Medical Journal* (May 13, 1989) Myra McClure and Thomas Schulz present an article on the "Origin of HIV." They quickly dispose of the idea that AIDS escaped from a germ warfare laboratory by stating, "Lack of supporting evidence precludes serious discussion of such a bizarre hypothesis. This review deals with the theories on the origin of HIV that are scientifically plausible."

Thus, medical science continues to ignore all the circumstantial evidence that strongly suggests AIDS originated as a biowarfare experiment. Most physicians steadfastly hold on to the illogical and improbable green monkey theory of AIDS. Likewise, the media remains silent, quickly dismissing the biowarfare issue as communist propaganda of the most malicious sort. And the National Academy of Sciences is silent on its cooperative role with the military in the development of secret biological weapons for mass killings.

In June 1989 my book, *AIDS AND THE DOCTORS OF DEATH: AN INQUIRY INTO THE ORIGIN OF THE AIDS EPIDEMIC*, was suppressed at the Fifth International AIDS Conference at Montreal, Canada. The book was being sold at an exhibit sponsored by the Highway Bookshop. An official of the World Health Organization (one of the sponsors of the Conference) put pressure on the owners of the bookstore to remove the book from their shelves. The booksellers were intimidated into complying with the official's request.

A magazine article on the incident appeared in *The Guide to the Gay Northeast* (July 1989). In an interview a WHO employee (who asked not to be named) characterized the book as "right wing bigotry" and claimed the book contained a "number of really weird suppositions." He was also quoted as saying, "We can't actually make them (the booksellers) take it off their shelves." The reporter, Bill Andriette, commented: "It is curious that the WHO felt so threatened by Cantwell's criticisms that they thought it best to suppress his book at Montreal. One wonders why they felt it necessary to protect those attending the conference, the people in the world presumably best informed about AIDS. The WHO must believe either that Cantwell's claims are powerfully convincing, or that those spearheading the global fight against this illness are highly gullible."

I had come far afield of my work with the cancer microbe. I was no longer surprised by the dogmatism and the arrogance of the scientific estabishment. The scientific world that could never "see" the cancer microbe could not be expected to "see" AIDS as covert biowarfare. I had penetrated the soul of medical science and I had found its heart of darkness.

For the past century the pharmaceutical industry has attempted to develop a drug and a vaccine cure for cancer. None has been found. Sadly, many of the same scientists who failed in the 70s War on Cancer are now the leaders in the War on AIDS. In 1979 there were a handful of AIDS cases; in 1989 over 100,000 U.S. cases were officially recorded. Most people are still complacent about the disease, and we are only just beginning to see the true horror of the AIDS holocaust.

Away from the eye of the public, the cancer establishment has clandestinely carried out the insane animal experiments that have finally produced the predicted, genetically engineered "super germ" — the AIDS virus that the immune system is powerless to destroy.

The cancer virologists and the genetic engineers are the new masters of life and death on the planet. A century after Pasteur's discovery of disease-producing germs, the biotechnical medical world has joined forces with power-hungry world leaders, and with the military biowarfare establishment, and with greedy drug companies, and even with terrorists. This newly interconnected group has the power to force a different kind of "final solution" onto the peoples of the world.

The biomedical establishment seeks to manipulate and control the gene formation of all living things. A genetically engineered mouse has already been created and patented at Harvard; and the geneticists are feverishly mapping out the entire "human genome." Not even Hitler could have imagined the genetically-controlled master and slave races that will be developed in future centuries.

A new kind of insanity is beginning. And it hides under the name of medical science. Its hallmark is the utter lack of a philosophical system of ethics and morality.

References:

1. **Cantwell AR Jr**: Bacteriologic investigation and

histologic observations of variably acid-fast bacteria in three cases of Kaposi's sarcoma. Growth 45:79-89, 1981.

2. **Cantwell AR Jr, and Lawson JW**: Necroscopic findings of pleomorphic, variably acid-fast bacteria in a fatal case of Kaposi's sarcoma. J Dermatol Surg Oncol 7: 923-930, 1981.

3. **Cantwell AR Jr**: Variably acid-fast bacteria in vivo in a case of reactive lymph node hyperplasia occurring in a young male homosexual. Growth 46: 331-336, 1982.

4. **Cantwell AR Jr**: Kaposi's sarcoma and variably acid-fast bacteria in vivo in two homosexual men. Cutis 32: 58-64, 68, 1983.

5. **Cantwell AR Jr**: Necroscopic findings of variably acid-fast in a fatal case of acquired immunodeficiency syndrome and Kaposi's sarcoma. Growth 47: 129-134, 1983.

6. **Cantwell AR Jr**: *AIDS and the Doctors of Death.* Aries Rising Press, Los Angeles, 1988.

7. **Jones JH**: *Bad Blood: The Tuskegee Syphilis Experiment.* The Free Press, New York, 1981.

8. **Piller C, and Yamamoto KR**: *Gene Wars: Military Control over the New Genetic Technologies.* Beach Tree Books, William Morrow, New York, 1988.

9. **Harris R, and Paxman J**: *A Higher Form of Killing.* Hill and Wang, New York, 1982.

10. **McClure HM, Keeling ME, Custer RP, et al**: Erythroleukemia in two infant chimpanzees fed milk from cows naturally infected with bovine C-

type virus. Cancer Research 34: 2745-2757, 1974.

11. **Fogarty International Center Proceedings N. 15**. Biological significance of histocompatibility antigens. Federation Proceedings 31: 1087-1104, 1972.

12. *Biohazards in Biological Research*. Cold Spring Harbor Laboratory, Cold Spring Harbor, New York, 1973.

13. **Melbye M, Biggar RJ, Ebbesen P, et al**: Seroepidemiology of HTLV-III antibody in Danish homosexual men: Prevalence, transmission, and disease outcome. Brit Med J 289: 573-575, 1984.

14. **Goedert JJ, Biggar RJ, Winn DM, et al**: Decreased helper T lymphocytes in homosexual men: Sexual contact in high-incidence areas for the acquired immunodeficiency syndrome. Amer J Epidemiol 121: 629-636, 1985.

15. **Carswell JW, Sewankambo N, Lloyd D, et al**: How long has the AIDS virus been in Uganda? Lancet 1: May 24, 1986, p1217.

16. **Goodfield G**: *Quest for the Killers*. Birkhauser, Boston, 1985.

17. **Chase A**: *Magic Shots*. William Morrow and Co., New York, 1982.

18. **Executive Intelligence Review,** February 15, 1986. (PO Box 17390, Washington, DC, 20041-0390)

CHAPTER FOURTEEN

The Old Physician

No matter how I try to deny it, I am now officially old. A few months ago I was stunned when a young cashier casually offered me a senior citizen discount movie ticket. I can hardly believe I have been a physician for over thirty years. In the mirror I curiously observe my slowly aging body. I find myself becoming more sympathetic toward my older patients, and I listen more attentively to their problems.

Sexual ennui and my lover's fear of AIDS have long since destroyed our lovemaking, and it is strange being in a platonic love relationship. In the past five years dozens of friends, acquaintances, and patients have died horribly of AIDS, and dozens more are ill and "positive" for the AIDS virus. The gay life of the 60s and 70s has turned into a living hell for many homosexual men living in big cities.

For persons concerned about AIDS, sex without a condom is unthinkable; and scientists warn that condoms may not always prevent AIDS. Not surprisingly, Roman Catholic bishops oppose the use of condoms. In a major policy statement issued in November 1989, the bishops stressed chastity as the only "morally correct and medically sure" way to prevent the fatal disease. We are witnessing the slow death of sex on the planet, and I cannot bear to think about sexuality in the 1990s as millions of people become infected with the AIDS virus.

As the powerful planets of Uranus, Saturn, and Neptune transit my Sun-sign of Capricorn, my life undergoes great change. These planets symbolize creativity and discovery; patience and responsibility; and idealism and inspiration. With this intense planetary force focused in my tenth house of career, I feel the challenging karmic and spiritual energies which impel me to share my cancer microbe experiences with others.

After so many years, part of me is weary of cancer microbe research. I yearn to rid my bookshelves, closets, and filing cabinets of decades-old papers and research data. I am burned out on medical science and I feel the need for a change, a new interest.

My disillusionment with the medical profession is complete. I am bored by the leading-lights of dermatology who ignore cancer microbe research and preoccupy themselves with Retin-A for wrinkles, minoxidil for baldness, and liposuction for fat deposits. I resent the government retrovirologists and the AIDS "experts" who cry for more research money, but who have no desire to investigate the cancer bacteria that are so damn simple to see in the damaged AIDS tissue. I abhor the "green monkey" AIDS science of Robert Gallo, the world's leading AIDS scientist who misidentifies his laboratory contaminants as "new" viruses and advises celibacy until an AIDS cure is found.

My heroes in cancer research are passing from the scene. Irene Diller is gone. Florence Seibert is well over ninety. Eleanor is in poor health. Georges Mazet, who I met in Nice in 1987, is elderly and blind. Lida Mattman is officially retired, but still teaches microbiology at Wayne State. At age 84, Virginia is frail but manages to keep active. When her husband Owen died in 1988, she was terribly depressed and lonely. However, she has since married a man thirty years younger, and has perked up considerably.

There is hope that cancer microbe research will continue in the future. Some of the followers of Wilhelm Reich are interested in popularizing his seminal studies on the origin of cancer. Recently one of my most important research papers on AIDS-related Kaposi's sarcoma (with six full-page photos of the cancer microbe) was published in the November 1988 issue of the *Journal of Orgonomy*[1]. The *Journal* is dedicated to preserving Reich's work, and publishes current research relevant to orgone energy.

In the same issue of the *Journal*, Richard Blasband MD has written a brilliant paper entitled, "Transformations in microbiological organisms." The paper relates Reich's cancer T-bacilli discoveries to the work of Antoine Bechamp, Virginia Livingston, and other cancer microbe scientists.

Blasband takes issue with Pasteur's dogma regarding the origin of life. He writes: "Nowhere is this blind acceptance of authority more evident that in medical science's rigid acceptance of Pasteur's declaration, in 1864, that living organisms arise from parental organisms like themselves. The facts, and there are many, demonstrate these alleged rules of biological life to be true only within a very limited range of nature. Indeed, the reality is quite the opposite: Viable microorganisms are constantly developing from such organic materials as moss, grass, and animal protein; and, once formed, they are capable of transformations into other forms ranging from the fungus, through the bacteria, to the virus. There is also evidence that they can arise from inorganic clays, limestone, carbon, and silicon."[2]

Reich's controversial, weather-control "cloudbusting" experimental work also continues in the hands of Richard Blasband, James DeMeo, and others. *Pulse of*

the Planet,[3] a new quarterly journal of the Orgone
Biophysical Research Laboratory, emphasizes that
Reich's discoveries of biological and atmospheric energy
are crucial for understanding the basic nature of the
massive environmental and social problems that are now
affecting the world.

It is possible, but not probable, that the cancer cures
of forgotten scientists will be revived and allowed to be
tested by the "authorities" in the cancer establishment.
Currently, there is renewed interest in the work of Royal
Raymond Rife (1888-1971). Rife built a special microscope powerful enough to demonstrate the virus forms of
the cancer microbe. He also invented an electromagnetic
frequency instrument which apparently cured cancer.
The American Medical Association took action against
Rife and succeeded in destroying his career and his
instruments that held so much promise for a cancer
cure. Rife's tragic story is chronicled in *THE RIFE
REPORT: THE CANCER CURE THAT WORKED*
by Barry Lynes and John Crane[4]. Barry Lynes has also
written *THE HEALING OF CANCER: THE CURES,
THE COVER-UPS AND THE SOLUTION NOW!*
(1989), a scathing indictment of the American Cancer
Society, the American Medical Association, the National
Cancer Institute, the Federal Drug Administration, and
the medical establishment. Lynes believes an organized
conspiracy exists that will never allow a cancer cure to
be developed[5].

The late Antoine Priore, an Italian engineer who
worked in France, is another forgotten genius who
invented an electromagnetic ray machine that was
successful in healing hopeless cancer patients. Like the
inventions of other scientists who attempted to cure
cancer by "unorthodox" and drug-free methods, Priore's

machine was doomed by the action of the biomedical establishment.

Priore's machine utilized "scalar magnetic" energy. Details of Priore's work can be found in Lieutenant Colonel Tom Bearden's book, *AIDS BIOLOGICAL WARFARE*[6]. Bearden's professional and military credentials are impeccible. He is an expert in air defense systems; technical intelligence; nuclear weapons employment; and antiradiation missile countermeasures. Bearden explains, in simple terms, the therapeutic uses of electromagnetic healing energy that hold so much promise for a cancer and AIDS cure. Unfortunately, medical research in this field of biophysics area has been vigorously suppressed by the government and the pharmaceutical establishment. Bearden concludes that the development of scalar electromagnetic technology must be our top priority in the fight against AIDS biological warfare. He cautions: "Ironically, this time our entire system — the government, the medical establishment, the scientific establishment, the universities — all are far too dogmatic, and have far too sluggish a response time, to offer any assistance at all. They are simply so 'out of it' that they don't know what's really happened."

Gaston Naessens is a French biologist who has perfected a powerful Rife-like microscope that utilizes ultraviolet and laser technology. In the 1950s, Naessens purportedly discovered a cancer cure (based on a serum made from the cancer microbe) which was confiscated by the French government. In a merciless trial, the French Ministry of Health prosecuted Naessens to the full extent of the law. Naessens now works in Canada.

Employing his special "Somatoscope" microscope, Naessens has uncovered a tiny (0.1 micron) energetic "elementary particle" that he calls a "somatid." The somatid is part of a life cycle of a pleomorphic microbe that Naessens has found in the body fluid and in the blood. He claims he has cultured somatids in his laboratory. Raymond Keith Brown MD has written favorably about Naessens research in *AIDS, CANCER AND THE MEDICAL ESTABLISHMENT*[7]. Color photographs of somatids in red blood cells are included in Brown's book. Naessen's somatids are undoubtedly related to Bechamp's microzymas, Reich's bions, and to certain growth phases of Virginia Livingston's pleomorphic cancer microbe.

In June 1989 Naessens was arrested and charged with practicing medicine without a license. He is accused of swindling the public with a quack treatment for cancer and AIDS. Naessens is awaiting trial in Quebec, and his case has become a "cause celebre." Some patients and physicians insist that Naessens is a miracle worker. Bernard Baril, a 33 year-old AIDS patient, developed an incurable cancer inside his mouth. His physicians told him there was nothing that could be done. Baril lost his job and became suicidal. After receiving Naessens "serum" for three weeks, his cancer disappeared. Other deathly ill AIDS patients have also benefited from Naessens therapy.

Dr. Augustin Roy, head of the Corporation profesionelle des medicins, has branded Naessens a quack. According to the *Montreal Gazette* (June 25, 1989), Roy has never visited Naessen's lab. When asked if the medical profession has officially investigated Naessen's claims, Roy said, "It's not our job." He further added, "A real scientist does not behave that way. A real scientist completes his studies, submits the results to analysis, does not hide his formula and, if he believes he's found something and wants to make it available to the public, has it approved by the proper government authorities."

A few scientists continue to research the pleomorphic forms of the tubercle bacillus, the acid-fast microbe intimately related to the cancer microbe. Tania Korsak, an elderly Belgian microbiologist, still avidly studies cell wall deficient forms of TB mycobacteria. When I visited her in Brussels in 1987 she presented me with magnificent color photos of these pleomorphic TB microbes. Some of these pictures were previously published in 1975 in the *ACTA Tuberculosea et Pneumologica Belgica*[8]. Dr. Korsak is currently studying a new growth form of mycobacteria that has never been recorded in the literature.

Although Tania's TB research is little known and unappreciated, I continue to be inspired by her observations. Tania has recently written: "The acid-fast rod form of the tubercle bacillus never develops alone in culture. As the acid-fast rods decompose and breakdown in the culture, the TB culture becomes a mixture of bacterial forms and virus forms and all the intermediate stages. The "coccoid forms" you have studied in AIDS and cancer are a part of the intermediate stage. *These coccoid forms are not staphylococci! All the laboratories identify them as such, but it's a mistake. They are viral forms — the famous filterable virus, searched for since the last century. The coccoid forms are not necessarily "acid-fast" like the tubercle bacillus. One can find blue (non-acid-fast) and red (acid-fast) cocci in the same culture at the same time*[9].

Few people understand the importance of Tania's observations. I understood because I had studied the bacteriology of scleroderma, cancer, AIDS, and dozens of other diseases "of unknown etiology." Sometimes the microbes were acid-fast and sometimes they weren't. When the microbes were cultured, they frequently looked like common "staphylococci." But if one observed the cocci over a period of time, they often changed into other forms totally unlike common staphylococci!

A knowledge of microbial pleomorphism, particularly of the tubercle bacillus, is indispensible for studying bacteria associated with cancer and AIDS. It is a continuing tragedy that microbiologists, pathologists, oncologists, dermatologists, and other physicians and researchers are not willing to investigate the microbe of cancer.

The AIDS holocaust and the urgent need for an AIDS cure may force government scientists to reinvestigate the cancer microbe and its role in various diseases. For several years, Dr. Shyh-Ching Lo has been studying a new, cancer-causing, "virus-like agent" that he discovered in AIDS and Kaposi's sarcoma. A recent *New York Native* article (November 13, 1989) claims Lo's virus may be a cell wall deficient bacterium. Charles Ortleb writes: "Sources famliar with AIDS research that is being conducted at the Armed Forces Institute of Pathology in Washington have told the *Native* that Dr. Shyh-Ling Lo will soon make public the nature of the agent he discovered three years ago in AIDS patients. Lo's agent, which he has called Virus-Like Infectious Agent (VLIA) in several papers will be identified as a mycoplasma, which is a form of bacteria that lacks a cell wall. The *Native* has also learned that Lo will name his agent *Mycoplasma incognitus*." (It will be interesting to see if Lo's relates his new "agent" to the cancer microbe — the hidden killer in AIDS).

Lo's research illustrates the important connection

between virology and bacteriology, a connection that is ignored in modern medical science. In artificially and arbitrarily separating various aspects of microbiology, medical science has created barriers that make it impossible to discover the infectious nature of cancer and the hidden microbe of AIDS. Virologists study viruses; and bacteriologists study bacteria. Virologists don't comprehend that viruses can originate from bacteria. And bacteriologists don't comprehend that bacteria can originate from viruses. And few physicians understand that "mycoplasmas" comprise the borderline stages between viruses and bacteria. It is pathetic that closed-minded scientists cannot see the vital interconnections between these branches of microbiology.

It is more than a quarter-century since I first examined Willa's painful nodules and looked into Reuben's tormented eyes. Willa and Reuben would have been surprised at the chain of events they started. They taught me so much and yet I still have not learned how to heal the diseases that plagued them.

Of course, I could impress them with all I had discovered about their hidden microbes, and I could explain how their microbes looked like the microbe of cancer. But if they asked me for a drug or a treatment, I would have to admit that I didn't know how to kill their microbes.

The most difficult thing in life is to learn how to heal. Students of metaphysics are taught that we are here on the planet for a purpose. Our purpose is to heal — and in order to heal others, we must first learn to heal ourselves. Perhaps my cancer microbe work has been a beginning in my healing.

As a physician and scientist I have learned the cancer

microbe is indestructible. And I have learned a little about the forces and the "conditions" (as Edgar Cayce would say) that propel the cancer microbe to activity.

Because the cancer microbe arises from life, it cannot be destroyed. It can only be transformed. Spiritual healers all teach the great importance of personal "transformation" in the healing process.

As an enigmatic killer and creator of life, the cancer microbe may be a symbol that reflects the paradoxical nature of our human psyche.

Within the realm of the cancer microbe lies the secrets of life. A life with no beginning and no end.

Scientists like Wilhelm Reich and Antoine Bechamp, and Virginia Livingston and Eleanor Alexander-Jackson, all recognized the immense power that resides within the cancer microbe: the power that exists within every living cell of every living creature in the universe.

Within the cancer microbe lies the indestructible force that contains the essence of healing.

It is written that He had the power to heal though the power of love. No drugs, no vaccines, no machines or gadgets, no surgery. Only love. Medical science would do well to investigate this power.

One day we will learn to harness this God-like force. And we will heal like He did.

But that is another story that must await another time.

References:

1. **Cantwell AR Jr, Blasband RA**: Bionous tissue degeneration in three patients with AIDS. Journal of Orgonomy 22: 220-226, 1988. (Orgonomic Publications, PO Box 490, Princeton, NJ 08542).

2. **Blasband RA**: Transformations in microbiological organisms. Journal of Orgonomy 22: 293-300, 1988.

3. **DeMeo J (Editor)**: Pulse of the Planet. Orgone Biophysical Research Laboratory, PO Box 1395, El Cerrito, CA 94530.

4. **Lynes B, Crane J**: *The Rife Report: The Cancer Cure That Worked*. Marcus Books, Toronto, Canada, 1987.

5. **Lynes B**: *The Healing of Cancer*. Marcus Books, 1989 (PO Box 327, Queensville, Ontario, Canada, L0G 1R0).

6. **Bearden TE**: *AIDS Biological Warfare*. Tesla Book Company, 1988 (PO Box 1649, Greenville, TX 75401)

7. **Brown RK**: *AIDS, Cancer and the Medical Establishment*. Robert Speller Publishers, New York, NY, 1986.

8. **Korsak T**: Occurrence of L-forms in a case of generalized mycobacteriosis due to mycobacterium scrofulaceum. Acta Tuberc Pneumol Belg 66: 445-469, 1975.

MICROPHOTOGRAPHS

The following 19 microphotographs illustrate various microscopic appearances of the "cancer microbe" in diseased tissue and in laboratory culture. The microscopic magnification of each photo is 1000 times.

Figure 1:   SCLERODERMA; rod-shaped bacteria in skin smear.

Figure 2:   SCLERODERMA; rod-shaped bacteria in skin.

Figure 3:   SCLERODERMA; coccoid bacteria in skin.

Figure 4:   SCLERODERMA; giant forms in skin.

Figure 5:   ACID-FAST BACTERIA cultured from scleroderma.

Figure 6.   SARCOID REACTION; coccoid bacteria in skin.

Figure 7:   LYMPHOMA; coccoid bacteria in lymph node.

Figure 8:   HODGKIN'S DISEASE; Russell body in lymph node.

Figure 9:   HODGKIN'S DISEASE; coccoid bacteria in skin.

Figure 10:   *Propionibacterium acnes* cultured from Hodgkin's disease.

Figure 11:   BREAST CANCER; coccoid bacteria in breast.

Figure 12:   *Staphylococcus epidermidis* cultured from breast cancer.

Figure 13:   INTERSTITIAL PNEUMONITIS (AIDS);
coccoid bacteria in lung.

Figure 14:   *Mycobacterium   avium-intracellulare*
cultured from interstitial pneumonitis.

Figure 15:   LYMPH NODE HYPERPLASIA (AIDS);
Russell bodies in lymph node.

Figure 16:   KAPOSI'S SARCOMA (AIDS); coccoid
bacteria in skin.

Figure 17:   IMMUNOBLASTIC SARCOMA (AIDS);
rod-shaped bacteria in skin.

Figure 18:   *Mycobacterium   avium-intracellulare*
cultured from immunoblastic sarcoma.

Figure 19:   BASAL CELL CARCINOMA; coccoid
bacteria in skin.

Figure 1

Diagnosis: Scleroderma

Tissue: Skin smear

A 37 year-old white man had scleroderma of the skin with ulcerations. A small portion of the skin near one of these ulcerations was removed and sent to the laboratory for culture of bacteria.

The skin specimen was ground-up in a special tissue grinder, and the material was subsequently stained with the Ziehl-Neelsen (acid-fast) stain. Tissue acid-fast stains are used to color and detect tuberculosis-type bacteria.

The photograph shows numerous acid-fast, red-stained, bacterial rods in the ground-up tissue smear. The appearance of this microbe in bacterial culture is shown in Figure 5. Figures 1-5 are all from the same case of scleroderma, described in the text as patient Reuben.

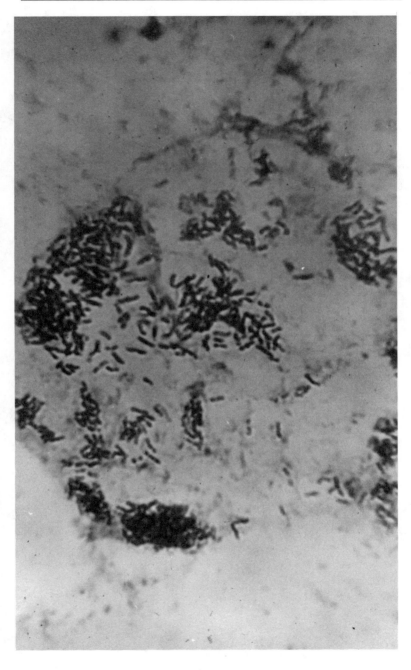

Figure 2

Diagnosis: Scleroderma

Tissue: Skin

A skin tissue section of scleroderma stained for acid-fast bacteria with the Fite-Faraco (acid-fast) stain. Arrows point to short, acid-fast, red-stained bacterial rods detected in the dermis portion of the skin. (Same case as Figure 1).

These rod-shaped, acid-fast bacteria are similar in size and shape to the acid-fast bacteria that were cultured from the diseased skin (Figure 5).

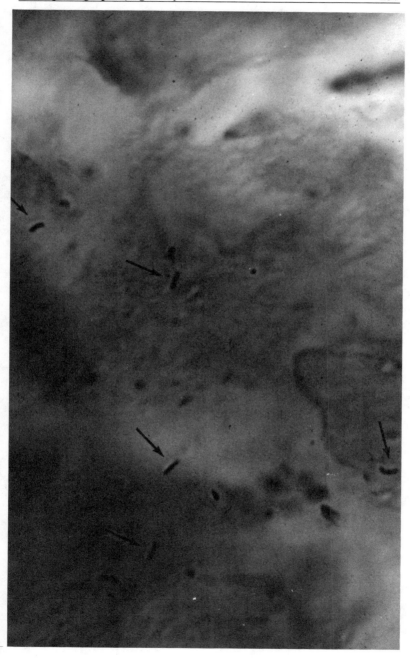

Figure 3

Diagnosis: Scleroderma
         Tissue: Skin

An acid-fast, Fite-Faraco stained tissue section of scleroderma skin showing numerous acid-fast, red-stained, round coccoid-shaped and granular microbial forms in the dermis portion of the skin.

These coccoid and granular forms are similar in size and shape to the coccus forms grown in culture (Figure 5.)

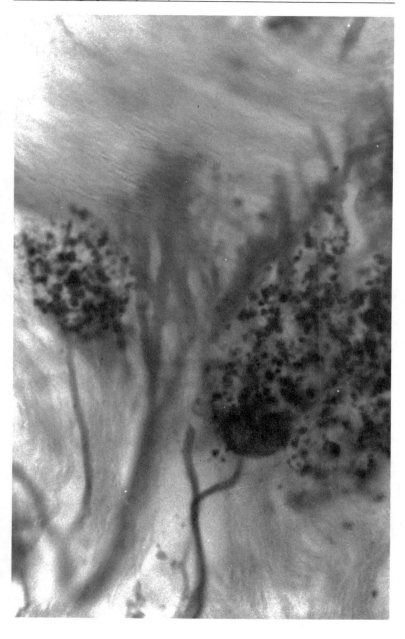

Figure 4

Diagnosis: Scleroderma
          Tissue: Skin

Large, balloon-like, giant round forms in the fatty portion (panniculus) of the skin in scleroderma. These giant forms are much larger than bacteria. The size and shape of these large forms resemble yeast and fungus-like organisms. They also resemble the Russell bodies pictured in Figures 8 and 15.

These forms were diagnosed by the pathologist as "fat degeneration." However, an alternative explanation is that these "large bodies" are growth forms of "cell wall deficient bacteria," known as "giant L forms." (Further details of these giant microbial forms can be found in Lida Mattman's *CELL WALL DEFICIENT FORMS*, CRC Press, 1974.)

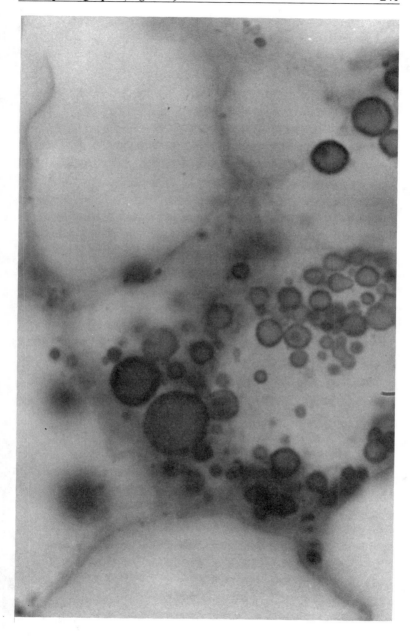

Figure 5

Subject: Acid-fast bacteria cultured from scleroderma

A tuberculosis-type microbe isolated from the skin of a scleroderma patient (Same case as Figures 1-4). The microbe is pleomorphic and appears in two distinct forms: 1) a non-acid- fast, blue-stained, round coccus form; 2) and an acid-fast, red- stained rod form. This photograph shows numerous tiny cocci. In the center of the photo arrows points to a group of red rods developing from the blue cocci.

The blue-stained coccus forms in culture are similar in size and shape to the coccoid forms detected in the skin of scleroderma (Figure 3).

The acid-fast, red-stained rod forms in culture are similar in size and shape to the acid-fast rod forms detected in the skin of scleroderma (Figure 2).

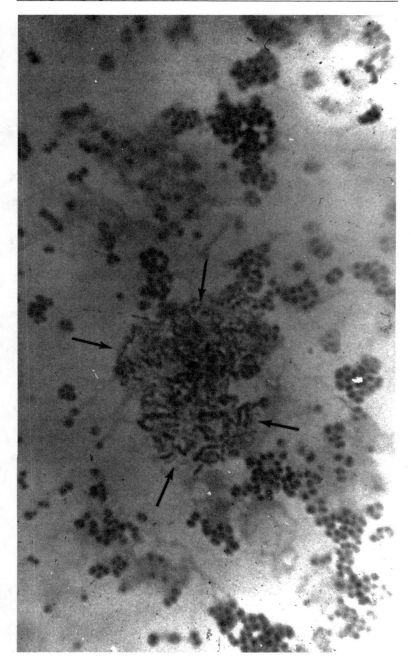

Figure 6

Diagnosis: Sarcoid reaction
            Tissue: Skin

One year before her diagnosis of lymphoma cancer, a 73 year-old white woman developed several facial inflammatory lesions interpreted by the pathologist as "sarcoid reaction." The cause of this reaction is unknown.

The pathologist could not detect microbes in the skin tissue sections. However, intensified Kinyoun-stained (acid-fast) sections revealed foci of acid-fast coccoid microbial forms in the dermis portion of the skin.

Similar-appearing coccoid-shaped microbial forms were also identified in the lymphoma cancer tissue (Figure 7).

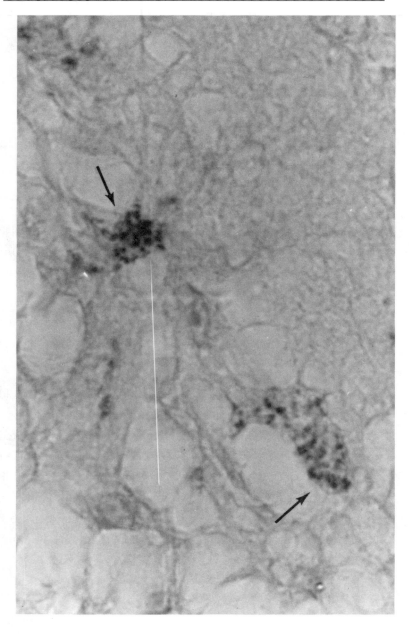

Figure 7

Diagnosis: Lymphoma

Tissue: Lymph node

A 73 year-old woman with "sarcoid reaction" (Figure 6) also developed enlarged lymph nodes of the neck and armpits. One of these nodes was removed for biopsy. The pathologist diagnosed malignant lymphoma, a form of cancer.

A Fite-stained, acid-fast section of the lymph node showed clumped, intracellular coccoid forms, consistent with "cancer microbes."

Similar shaped coccoid forms were identified in the "sarcoid reaction" (Figure 6). Sarcoid reactions are found in "sarcoidosis," an inflammatory disease that is thought to be possibly related to tuberculosis. Sarcoid tissue reactions can also occur in cancer patients who do not have sarcoidosis. The peculiar relationship between sarcoid reaction and cancer is unknown. However, microbes resembling "cancer microbes" can be found in both cancer and "sarcoid reaction," as illustrated in this woman's case.

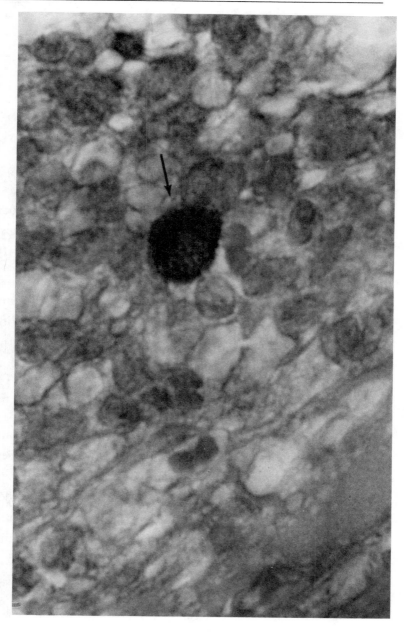

Figure 8

Diagnosis: Hodgkin's Disease
                   Tissue: Lymph node

An elderly white woman developed an enlarged lymph node of the neck. The diseased gland was removed and the pathologist diagnosed Hodgkin's Disease, a malignant form of cancer. Thirty years previously she had breast cancer.

The tissue sections were stained for bacteria by use of a Gram stain, a commonly used stain for the detection of bacteria. With this stain, numerous Russell bodies were detected within the cancerous lymph node. Russell's bodies were discovered a century ago by the Scottish pathologist, William Russell. He believed the bodies represented the "parasite of cancer."

At present, the exact origin and nature of Russell bodies are unknown. Athough they are considered non-microbial, Russell bodies bear a strong resemblance to giant forms of "cell wall deficient bacteria," known as "large bodies." The Russell bodies in this case of Hodgkin's Disease are similar to the Russell bodies observed in an inflamed lymph node in AIDS (Figure 15). They are also similar to the "large bodies" seen in scleroderma (Figure 4).

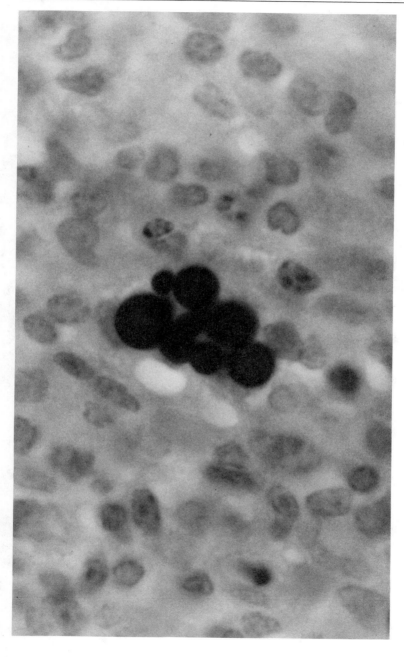

Figure 9

Diagnosis: Hodgkin's Disease
            Tissue: Skin

An acid-fast, Fite-stained tissue section of skin from the face showing Hodgkin's Disease, a form of cancer. The arrows point to a collection of coccoid forms in the dermis portion of the skin.

These tiny, coccoid and granular forms are similar in size and shape to the coccoid and granular forms of *Propionibacterium acnes*, which were cultured from the cancerous skin lesion (Figure 10).

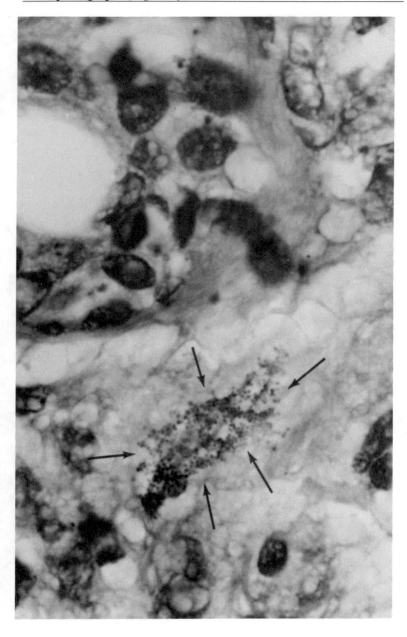

Figure 10

Subject: *Propionibacterium acnes* cultured from Hodgkin's Disease

A microphotograph of *Propionibacterium acnes* cultured from the facial skin lesion of Hodgkin's Disease pictured in Figure 9. *Propionibacterium acnes* is also known as *Corynebacterium acnes*, a common skin microbe. The organism is pleomorphic and exists in two forms: rods and granules.

In addition to the rod forms, species of corynebacteria cultured from cancerous and inflammatory diseases may also appear as coccus forms. Corynebacterial (diphtheroid) bacteria of this mixed type are known as "coccobacilli."

P. acnes is not an acid-fast microbe, although the corynebacteria are closely related to the acid-fast mycobacteria. An unusual feature of this microbe in this culture is that a few of the rods were acid-fast and stained red. The large arrows point to the rods forms of *P. acnes*. The small arrows point to the tiny "granules," which are acid-fast.

The "granules" in this culture of *P. acnes* are the same size and shape as the coccoid forms detected in the dermis portion of the skin lesion of Hodgkin's Disease pictured in Figure 9.

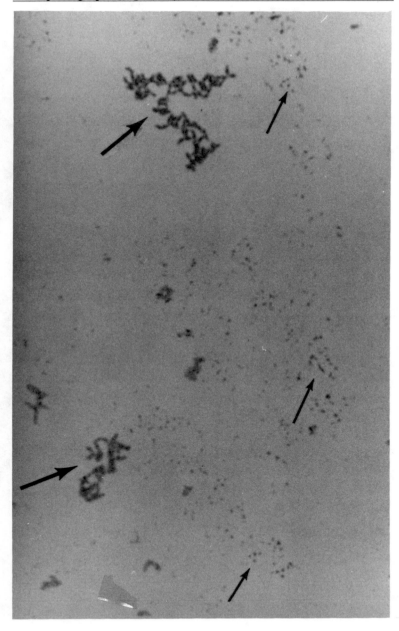

Figure 11

Diagnosis: Breast cancer
          Tissue: Breast

An acid-fast, intensified Kinyoun stained tissue section of a cancerous breast showing two areas of coccoid microbes. The small arrow points to coccoid forms appearing within a cell (intracellular). The large arrow points to coccoid forms outside the cell (extracellular).

The size and shape of these coccoid forms are similar to the coccus forms of *Staphylococcus epidermidis* cultured from the breast cancer when it spread to the skin (Figure 12).

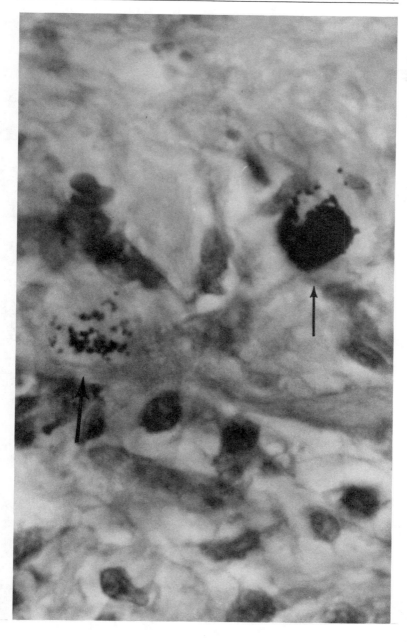

Figure 12

Subject: *Staphylococcus epidermidis* cultured from breast
cancer

An acid-fast stained smear of *Staphylococcus epidermidis*
cultured from a breast cancer tumor that spread to the skin.
The coccus forms of the microbe are similar in size and shape
to the intracellular and extracellular coccoid forms identified
in the patient's original tumor (Figure 11).

In addition to the non-acid-fast (blue-stained) cocci, there are
also acid-fast (red-stained) "spicules" and "filaments." The
arrows point to these filaments. Acid-fast spicules and filaments
arising from coccus forms of the cancer microbe have been
described and illustrated by Virginia Livingston and Eleanor
Alexander-Jackson (An experimental approach to the treatment
of neoplastic disease. Journal of the American Medical Women's
Association, Volume 20, pages 858-866, 1965.)

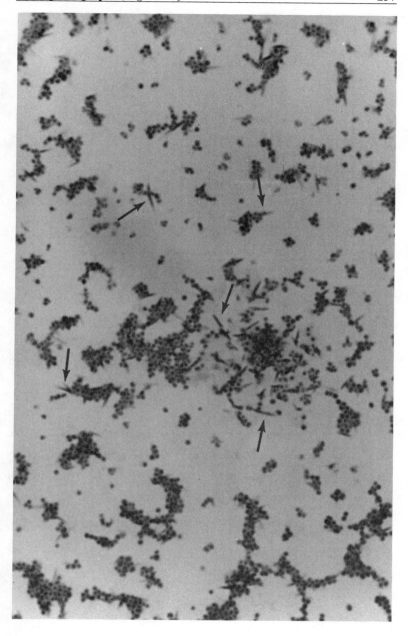

Figure 13

Diagnosis: Interstitial pneumonitis, AIDS
                    Tissue: Lung

A Fite-stained (acid-fast) section of lung tissue taken from a 29 year-old gay man with AIDS and pneumonia. The pathologist's diagnosis of the lung tissue is "interstitial pneumonitis," an inflammation of the lung "of unknown etiology." No microbes were detected by the pathologist.

In the center of the photograph is a focus of tiny coccoid forms revealed by the acid-fast stain. These forms are similar in size and shape to the coccus forms of *Mycobacterium avium-intracellulare*, which were cultured from the "bronchial washings" of the patient's inflamed lungs (Figure 13).

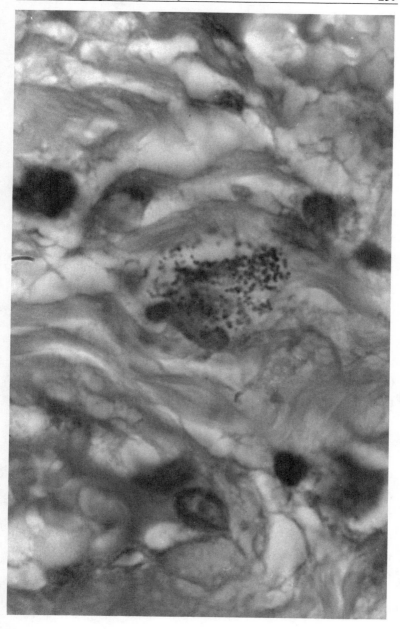

Figure 14

Subject: *Mycobacterium avium-intracellulare* cultured from interstitial (lung) pneumonitis

Mycobacterium avium-intracellulare was cultured from the bronchial (windpipe) washings of a gay man with AIDS and "interstitial pneumonitis."

M. avium-intracellulare exists in two forms: a rod-shaped form and a coccus form. In this culture the rods were acid-fast; the cocci were non-acid-fast.

The coccus forms of *M. avium-intracellulare* are similar in size and shape to the coccoid forms detected in the lung pneumonia (Figure 13). This similarity suggests that the coccoid forms in the lung actually represent hidden and unrecognized infection with *M. avium-intracellulare*.

M. avium-intracellulare can cause tuberculosis and other diseases. Pathologists look for acid-fast rod forms in order to diagnose infection with this microbe. Pathologists do not accept tissue non-acid-fast coccoid forms of mycobacteria as a diagnostic sign of infection with these microbes. In fact, all the diseases presented in this series of photographs with coccoid forms in the tissue were considered "negative" for microbes, according to the pathologists.

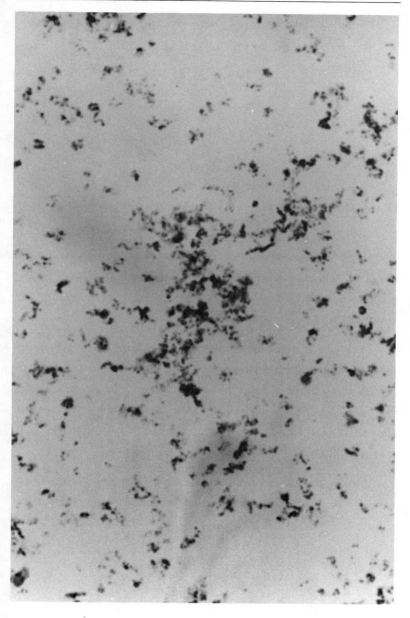

Figure 15

Diagnosis: Reactive lymph node hyperplasia, AIDS

Tissue: Lymph node

A 44 year-old gay man with AIDS developed enlarged lymph nodes of the neck, armpits and groin. One of these diseased nodes was removed. The pathologist diagnosed "non-specific hyperplasia" of the node. No microbes were identified.

A Gram-stain for bacteria showed numerous intra- and extracellular Russell bodies. The curved arrow points to Russell bodies developing inside a cell (intracellular). The straight arrow points to larger Russell bodies which have apparently shattered the cell and appear to be developing outside the cell (extracellular).

Russell bodies were originally described as the "parasite of cancer." Russell bodies in Hodgkin's Disease are pictured in Figure 8.

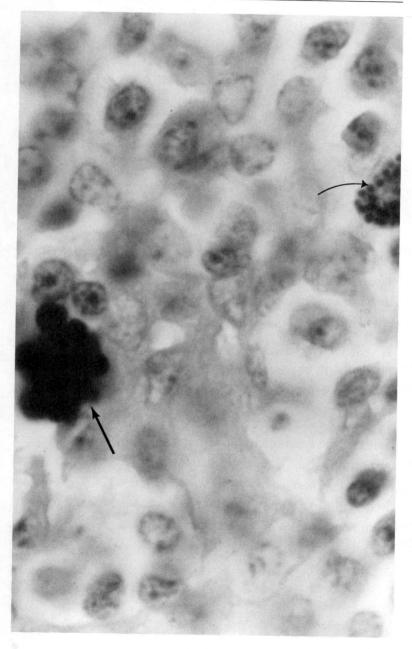

Figure 16

Diagnosis: Kaposi's Sarcoma (AIDS)

Tissue: Skin

A Fite-stained, acid-fast tissue section of a skin tumor of Kaposi's sarcoma of the leg. Arrows point to numerous coccoid forms that are present in the tumor area. The patient was a 36 year-old, white gay man.

A year later he developed an "immunoblastic sarcoma" of the face (Figure 17) from which a pleomorphic, tuberculosis-type microbe (*Mycobacterium avium-intracellulare*) was cultured (Figure 18).

The coccoid forms pictured here in the Kaposi's sarcoma tumor are similar in size and shape to the coccus forms of *Mycobacterium avium-intracellulare* (Figure 18). This suggests that acid-fast rod forms of tuberculous bacteria may originate from non-acid-fast coccoid forms in tissue.

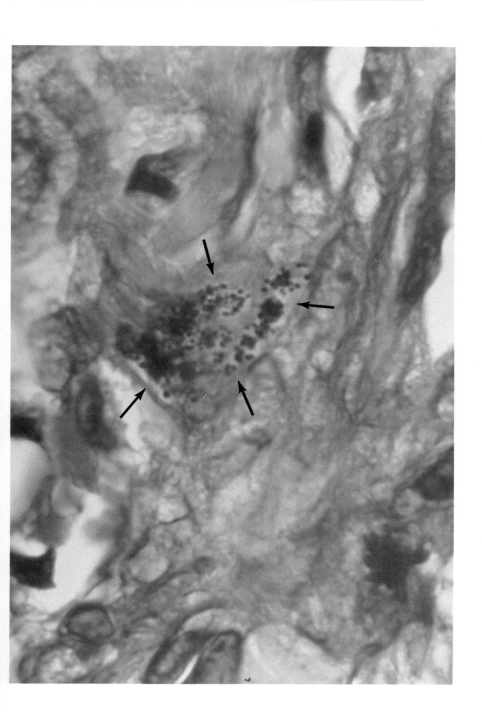

Figure 17

Diagnosis: Immunoblastic sarcoma (AIDS)

Tissue: Skin

A Fite-stained, acid-fast tissue microscopic section of a skin tumor of "immunoblastic sarcoma" located on the face of a 36 year-old man dying of AIDS.

The arrows point to three typical rod-shaped, red-stained, acid-fast bacteria present in the tumor area. A pleomorphic microbe, *Mycobacterium avium-intracellulare*, was cultured from the tumor (Figure 18).

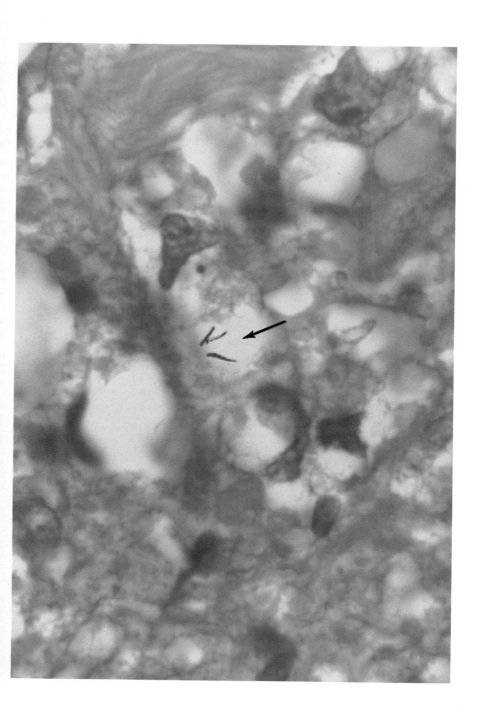

Figure 18

Subject: *Mycobacterium avium-intracellulare* cultured from immunoblastic sarcoma

Mycobacterium avium-intracellulare cultured from an "immunoblastic sarcoma" tumor on the face of a 36 year-old white gay man dying of AIDS.

This microbe is pleomorphic and exists in two forms. One form is a red-stained, acid-fast rod form. The other is a non- acid-fast, blue-stained coccus form (arrows).

The acid-fast rod form of this tuberculosis-causing microbe is similar in size and shape to the acid-fast rods identified in the immunoblastic sarcoma tumor from which it was cultured (Figure 17). The coccus form of the microbe is also similar in size and shape to the coccoid forms present in the Kaposi's sarcoma tumor of the same man (Figure 16).

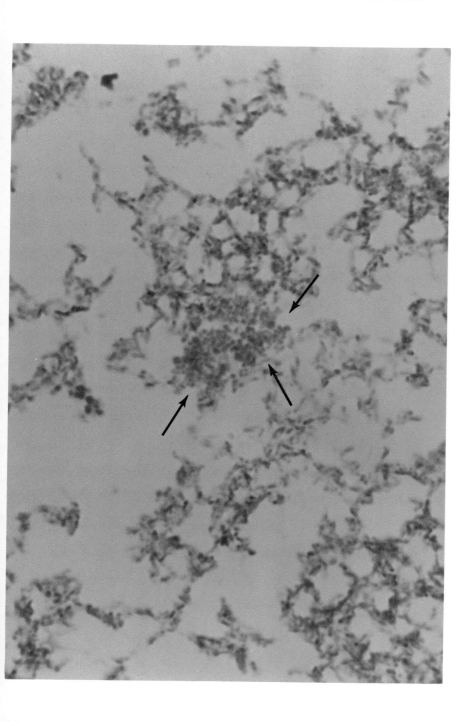

Figure 19

Diagnosis: Basal cell carcinoma
              Tissue: Skin

Basal cell carcinoma of the skin is the most common form of cancer in white-skinned people. It is a rare cancer in dark-skinned people. In most cases, chronic sun damage precedes the development of this form of cancer.

In the center of the photograph arrows point to a small collection of purple-stained coccoid forms. Coccoid forms frequently appear in and around the tumor cells of this cancer. The size and shape of these coccoid forms are similar in appearance to the coccus forms of staphylococci and corynebacteria (coccobacilli), which can be cultured from skin cancer.

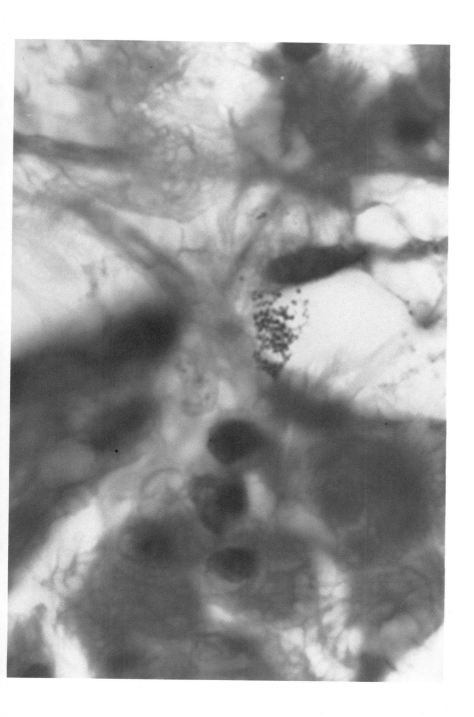

Conclusion

The "cancer microbe" can be detected in cancer and other diseases by staining the tissue with an acid-fast stain. Ordinarily, the identification of intracellular and extracellular "coccoid forms" suggests the presence of the cancer microbe. There is no single or specific appearance of the cancer microbe. As these photos attest, the microbe is pleomorphic and may appear in tissue and in culture in more than one form.

In order to understand the significance of the microbe it is necessary to carefully study the work of cancer microbiologists, such as Virginia Livingston, Eleanor Alexander-Jackson, Irene Diller, Florence Seibert, and others.

The possible "origin" of the cancer microbe can be found in the experimental data, writings, and theories of scientists like Antoine Bechamp and Wilhelm Reich.

In the continuing search for an underlying "cause" for cancer and other chronic illnesses of man, it would seem prudent for adventurous medical scientists to begin a thorough investigation into the teachings and claims of the cancer microbe scientists.

Subject Index

A

Aboriginals 145-149
acid-fast bacteria (also see mycobacteria) 37-40, 44-48, 50-51, 58-63, 65-66, 71-76, 85, 91, 99, 103, 105, 110, 234, 236, 238, 242, 260, 264, 266, 268
acid-fast stain 37, 44, 59-61, 103, 110, 234, 238, 242, 244, 246, 250, 252, 254, 256, 258, 260, 264, 266, 268, 272
acquired immune deficiency syndrome (see AIDS)
AIDS 44, 64, 73, 92, 114, 122-123, 137, 142-143, 150, 185-192, 199, 201, 203-217, 221-223, 225-229, 258, 260, 262, 264, 266, 268
— in African Blacks 186-187, 189-191, 204-207, 209-214
— sex and AIDS 187-189, 204-206
— statistics 216
amoebae 132, 163-165, 170
amoeboid parasites 106
amyotrophic lateral sclerosis 30
animal cancer 59, 106, 170, 198
animal cancer viruses 198-199, 212
animal experiments 98-99, 191
astrology 53-54, 202
atypical mycobacteria 38, 46-47, 51
autopsy studies 40, 49-50, 93-94, 110, 114, 123, 192

B

bacteria 12-13, 59, 81, 92, 109-113, 122, 134-136, 143, 145, 165-166, 168, 186, 204, 223, 228-229

bacteriologists 112, 114, 229
bacteriology 62, 71, 111, 229
basal cell cancer 270
biological warfare 190-198, 211, 215, 225
bionous degeneration 169
bions 169-172, 176-177, 226
Blacks 189-192, 199, 206-209, 213
blastomycetes 106
blood 62, 75, 78, 81, 110, 144, 171, 188-189, 201-202, 211
body armoring 159
bone marrow 62
bovine leukemia virus 190
bovine visna virus 190, 212-213
breast cancer 100, 103-104, 108, 122, 248, 254, 256

C

calf serum 212-213
cancer 11-15, 44, 58-64, 67-68, 73-75, 77-82, 85-86, 93, 97, 99-100, 143, 150, 152, 155-156, 166-172, 176, 178, 200, 224-226, 228-229, 272
cancer coccidia 106
cancer establishment 63, 78, 217
cancer microbe (also see mycobacteria, Staphylococcus epidermidis) 11-15, 60-64, 67-68, 74, 77-83, 85-86, 100, 103-110, 114-116, 122-124, 131, 137-138, 142, 150-151, 186-187, 205, 222-223, 226-230, 272
cancer parasites 105-108, 248, 262
cancer viruses 12, 61
cell wall deficient bacteria 76, 92, 99, 104, 106, 113, 142, 228, 240, 248

chemotherapy 115
chickens 59, 74, 80
chimpanzees 198, 201
chromatin granules 131
classification of microbes 38-40,
    65, 111-112, 142, 163
cloud busting 179, 223
coccobacilli 65, 91, 98, 104, 111,
    252, 270
coccus 61, 63-67, 71-73, 92, 104,
    108-109, 111-112, 132, 134, 142,
    227, 238, 242, 244, 246, 250, 252,
    254, 256, 258, 260, 264, 268, 270,
    272
connective tissue disease 43
contaminants 12, 44, 51, 64, 106,
    110, 112, 166, 189, 207, 209-213
corynebacteria 72-73, 81, 91, 111-
    112, 252, 270
Corynebacterium acnes (see Pro-
    pionibacterium acnes)

D
Danish gay study 203
dermatologists 59, 64, 91-92, 113,
    222, 228
diet 85
diphtheroids 65, 67, 72, 112, 252
drug addicts 189

E
electromagnetic frequency instru-
    ment 224-225
emotional plague 159
epidemiologists 96, 200-201, 203-
    204

F
fermentation 127, 129-131, 143
fungi 38, 46-47, 49, 67, 73, 78, 104,
    109, 185, 223, 240

G
gay men (see homosexuals)
genetic engineering 190, 195, 199,
    217
geneticists 217
genocide 193
germ theory of disease 128, 133-

134, 145, 148-149, 151, 166
globoid forms 63, 71, 75, 104
gonorrhea 96, 201
Gram stain 248, 262
granules 38, 63, 65, 71-73, 91-92,
    104, 170, 238, 250, 252
green monkey theory of AIDS 189-
    190, 208-210, 213, 222
guinea pigs 59, 72, 74

H
Haiti 186-187, 189
Hansen's disease (see leprosy)
hematologists 113
hematoxylin bodies 113
hematoxylin-eosin stain 37
hemophiliacs 188
hepatitis 96, 213
hepatitis B vaccine 191, 201-203,
    210-211
herpes 96
histologists 60
Hodgkin's disease 73, 104, 110,
    248, 250
holistic medicine 121
homosexuality 25, 29, 53, 189
homosexuals 25, 94-97, 104, 122,
    185-187, 190-191, 195, 200-206,
    210-211, 216, 221, 258, 260, 264,
    266, 268
human biological warfare exper-
    iments 192-194
human cancer experiment 108
human choriogonadotropic hor-
    mone (HCG) 115-116
human T-cell leukemia/lymhoma
    virus 188
human T-cell lymphotropic virus
    188

I
immune system 115, 122, 143, 188,
    199
immunoblastic sarcoma 264, 266,
    268
immunoglobulins 106
infectious disease specialists 113,
    214

interstitial pneumonitis 258, 260

J

K

Kaposi's sarcoma 104, 122, 185-187, 203-206, 223, 264, 268
kitten experiment 136
Koch's postulates 134-135

L

large bodies 92, 97, 104, 113, 240
legionnaire's disease 204
leprosy 11-13, 38, 46-47, 50, 59, 75-77, 105
leukemia 81, 110, 143, 188, 199
L forms 76, 240
little bodies 131-132, 138
lupus erythematosus 43, 110-111, 113
lymphoma 99, 122, 188, 244, 246

M

mast cell granules 91-92
medical establishment 63, 79, 109, 138, 156, 168, 208, 224
metaphysics 229
mice experiments 40, 75-76, 78, 108
microbiologists 58, 61-62, 64, 66-68, 72, 76, 82, 109-111, 113, 134, 228, 279
microbiology 47, 56-57, 66-67, 74, 76, 79, 92, 111-112, 116, 130, 134, 151, 163, 222
micrococcus 81
microscopes 60-61, 75, 79, 106, 127, 164, 172, 182, 225
microscopists 58, 60
microsomes 131
microzymas 129, 131-138, 142-144, 148, 150-152, 155, 226
molecular granulations 131
Much's granules 72, 92
mycobacteria 37-38, 45-46, 64, 71, 75-76, 81, 227, 260
mycobacteriologists 72
Mycobacterium avium-intracellulare 258, 260, 264, 266, 268
Mycobacterium fortuitum 50-51

Mycobacterium leprae 38, 46, 76
Mycobacterium tuberculosis 37, 46, 71-74, 134-135
Mycoplasma incognitus 228
mycosis fungoides 104

N

Nocardia 46, 49
nutrition 146-147

O

oncologists 113, 172, 228
Oranur experiment 177-178
orgastic potency 157
orgone accumulator 172, 176, 179-180
orgone energy 158-159, 163, 169, 171, 175-177, 179, 183

P

panniculitis 38-40, 48, 240
panniculus 38
pansclerotic morphea 111
parasitic bodies 106
parasitic theory of cancer 107
pathologists 38, 44, 59, 61-62, 85, 91-92, 103, 113-114, 228
penicillin 192
plasma cells 106
pleomorphism, bacterial 61, 65-67, 72-76, 81, 91, 93, 98-99, 104, 106-107, 109, 111-113, 149, 226-228, 242, 252, 266, 268, 272
pleuropneumonia-like organisms (PPLO) 76
Pneumocystis carinii pneumonia 185, 198
precancer 115, 171
Progenitor cryptocides 67, 115, 137-138, 142
Propionibacterium acnes 98, 250, 252
protozoa 163, 165, 170, 172
pseudoscleroderma 97-98

Q

R

radiation therapy 115
rheumatoid arthritis 43

rods, bacterial 59, 61, 63, 65-67,
    71-74, 76, 81, 104, 107-109, 111,
    132, 134, 234, 236, 242, 252, 260,
    266, 268
Rous sarcoma virus 80
Russell bodies 106, 113, 240, 248,
    262

S

sarcoidosis 73, 97-99, 114, 244,
    246
sarcoma 80
scalar magnetic energy 225
scintillating corpuscles 131
sclerobacillus Wuerthele-Caspe
    60, 67
scleroderma 40-41, 43-48, 50-51,
    54-60, 64-68, 74-75, 85, 90-94,
    97-98, 110-114, 150, 234, 236,
    238, 240, 242
scurvy 145
sexually transmitted diseases (see
    venereal disease)
skin cancer 122, 270
smallpox vaccine 190, 212-214
sperm cells 115-116, 132
spicules 256
spontaneous regeneration 127-129
spores 107-109
sporozoons 106
staphylococci 67, 72-73, 81, 91,
    98, 104, 110-112, 227-228, 270
Staphylococcus epidermidis 64,
    98, 103, 110, 254, 256
streptococci 110
Streptomyces coelicolor 38
syphilis 11-12, 96, 105, 191-192

T

T-bacilli 155-156, 165, 168-172,
    223
tubercle bacillus (see Mycobac-
    terium tuberculosis)
tuberculosis 11-12, 36-39, 44-48,
    51, 54-57, 59, 68, 71-76, 80-81,
    90-92, 97-99, 105-106, 110, 112,
    134-135, 147, 157, 227-228, 264,
    268

tuberculosis virus 72, 227
Tuskegee experiment 191-192

U

uveitis 97-98

V

vaccines 78, 80, 86, 109, 143, 146-
    149, 190-191, 199, 201, 210-214
vaccinia virus 190
venereal disease 27, 28, 192, 200
vesicles 164-165, 170
vibrionen evolution 132, 142
virologists 172, 187, 198, 217, 229
viruses 12, 61, 80, 91, 122, 143,
    151, 213, 224, 227-229
visna virus 190
vitamin C 145-147
vitamins 86

W

X

Y

yeast-like forms 67, 104, 107, 112,
    132, 137, 240

Z

zooglear matrix 72, 74-75, 92

Index of Proper Names

A

Abbott Laboratories 77
ACTA TUBERCULOSEA ET PNEUMOLOGICA BELGICA 227
Alexander-Jackson, Eleanor 62, 68, 71-80, 82, 85-86, 92, 155, 182, 222, 230, 272
Allen, Roy 60-62, 79
A HIGHER FORM OF KILLING 194
AIDS AND THE DOCTORS OF DEATH 191, 215
AIDS BIOLOGICAL WARFARE 225
AIDS, CANCER AND THE MEDICAL ESTABLISHMENT 226
AIDS: THE MYSTERY AND THE SOLUTION 123, 142, 156
American Assn for the Advancement of Science 78
American Cancer Society 77, 85-86, 123, 224
AMERICAN JOURNAL OF MEDICAL SCIENCES 62
American Medical Assn 79, 122-123, 224
AMERICAN MEDICAL NEWS 122
AMERICAN REVIEW OF TU-BERCULOSIS 71
Anderson, John A 62
Andriette, Bill 216

ANNALS OF THE NEW YORK ACADEMY OF SCIENCES 82
ARCHIVES OF DERMATOL-OGY 40, 48, 85, 91, 93, 97, 112
Association for Research and Enlightenment (A.R.E.) 55
Averill, Roy 57

B

BAD BLOOD 192
Baker, Ellsworth 181-182
Baril, Bernard 226
Bastian, Henry Charleton 128-129
Bearden, Tom 225
Bechamp, Antoine 57, 123-126, 128-138, 141-145, 149-153, 155, 223, 226, 230, 272
BECHAMP OR PASTEUR? 123-124, 130
Becker, Sam 33-36
Berke, Meyer 33
Beinhauer, L 73, 98
Black, Francis 200
Blasband, Richard 223
Boadella, David 178
BRITISH MEDICAL JOURNAL 108, 215
British Museum Library 141
Brodkin, Eva 59-60
Brown, Helene 123
Brown, Raymond Keith 226
Bryant, Anita 96
Buchanan, George 108

C

CA—A CANCER JOURNAL FOR CLINICIANS 86
CANCER, A NEW BREAKTHROUGH 63, 79
Cancer Control Society 121-123
Cantwell Sr, Alan R 17, 19-20, 29-30, 87-88
Cantwell, Howard Danforth 17, 34, 87-88, 95
Cantwell, Frances Louise (mother) 17-18, 29-30, 88, 94-95
Cantwell, Frances Louise (sister) 17, 88
Caspe, Joseph 60
Cayce, Edgar 54-57, 121, 150, 230
CELL WALL DEFICIENT FORMS 92, 240
Centers for Disease Control (CDC) 192, 204, 205
Central Intelligence Agency (CIA) 194
CHARACTER ANALYSIS 158
Chase, Allen 213
Chatterjee, BR 76
Columbia University 201
COMPTES RENDUS 125, 129
Cooper, Judy 53
Cornell Medical College 62, 71, 74-75
Cornell University 18-20, 26
Craggs, Eugenia 37-40, 44-48, 51, 53, 64
Crane, John 224
Crawford, S 98

D

Dafoe, Roy Allen 17-18
Damon Runyan Fund 77
DeMeo, James 223
D'Eramo, James 204-205
DERMATOLOGICA 94, 98
Dettman, Glen 137-138, 141, 146, 149
Dettman, Ian 138
Diller, Irene 77-78, 81-82, 85, 222, 272
Dionne quintuplets 17-18

E

EDGAR CAYCE HANDBOOK FOR HEALTH 56
EDGAR CAYCE ON HEALING 56
Essex, Myron (Max) 206, 209-210
EVERY SECOND CHILD 145, 148
EVOLUTION AND THE ORIGIN OF LIFE 128
EXECUTIVE INTELLIGENCE REVIEW 214
Ewing, James 107

F

Federal Drug Administration (FDA) 176, 178-180, 224
FEDERATION PROCEEDINGS 199
Fisher, LW 73
Fogh, Jorgen 86
Fontes, A 72
Fort MacArthur Army Hospital, CA, 29, 31, 33-34
Fort Sam Houston, TX, 26
Foxman, Stuart 18
Francisco Moragas Antituberculosis Institute, Barcelona 98
French Academy of Science 125, 128-129, 131, 133, 136
Freud, Sigmund 157-158
FUNCTION OF THE ORGASM (1927) 161
FUNCTION OF THE ORGASM (1942) 159

G

Gallo, Robert 187, 204-207, 209, 214, 222
GENE WARS 193
Glover, TJ 108-109
Goodfield, June 210
Gordon, Ruth 38, 50
Grote, J 212
GROWTH 98, 123
GUIDE TO THE GAY NORTHEAST 216

Gullberg, E 98

H
Hallberg, V 98
Hansen, Gerhard 105
Harris, Robert 194
Harvard Medical School 206, 209-210
Hillier, James 61-62, 75-76, 79
Holiday, Billie 22-23
Hsu, Su-Ming 106
Hume, Ethel Douglas 123-125, 130-131

I
Institute for Cancer Research, Philadelphia, 77
International Academy of Preventive Medicine 148
INTERNATIONAL JOURNAL OF DERMATOLOGY 99, 112
INTERNATIONAL JOURNAL OF LEPROSY 76
Ishii, Shiro 193-194

J
Jones, James H 192
Jones, Jim 202
Jones, Joyce E 110-111
JOURNAL OF DERMATO-LOGIC SURGERY AND ONCOLOGY 103-104
JOURNAL OF ORGONOMY 223
JOURNAL OF THE AMERICAN WOMEN'S ASSOCIATION 256
JOURNAL OF THE MEDICAL SOCIETY OF NEW JERSEY 60
JOURNAL OF THE ROYAL SOCIETY OF MEDICINE (London) 212

K
Kanki, Phyllis 209-210
Kaposi, Moriz 186
Kelso, Dan 64-66, 91, 98, 100, 103-104, 110-111, 186
Kennedy, John F 35

Klein, R 106
Knafelc, Dorothy 141-144, 148
Knafelc, Julian 141
Koch, Robert 105, 134-135
Kolokerinos, Archie 145-149
Korsak, Tania 227
Krieger, Lisa 123
Kupsinel, Roy 123-137

L
LaRouche, Lyndon 214
LeCount, ER 106
Lee Foundation, Milwaukee 124
Leitch, Archibald 107-108
Leverson, Montague 124, 130
Levine, Martin P 192
LIFE 77-78
Lindenberg, Elsa 162, 168-169
Livingston, Afton 58
Livingston, Virginia Wuerthele-Caspe 58-64, 66-68, 74-75, 77-80, 82, 85-85, 91, 115-116, 121-122, 142, 155, 182, 187, 190, 222, 230, 256, 272
LONDON TIMES 214-215
Long Beach State University, CA 40, 48
Los Angeles Metropolitan Dermatologic Society 48
LOS ANGELES TIMES 128, 208-209
Lo, Shyh-Chung 228
Lynes, Barry 224

M
MAGIC SHOTS 214
Mansfield, Richard 50
Mattman, Lida 92-93, 103, 110, 222, 240
Mazet, Georges 110, 222
McClure, Myra 215
McGarey, Bill 55-56
McGarey, Gladys 55
Mellon, Ralph 73, 98
Merck Company 210-211
Merck, George 211
Mercy Hospital, San Diego 23-24

Mermod, Camille 59-60
Metropolitan General Hospital,
   New York City 22
Milk, Harvey 202
Mitsuoka, TY 98
MONITEUR SCIENTIFIQUE
   124-125
Montagnier, Luc 205-207
MONTREAL GAZETTE 226
Moscone, George 202
Morrison, A Cressy Memorial
   Prize 75
Much, Hans 72
Muni, Paul 147

N
Naessens, Gaston 225-226
National Academy of Science 197,
   215
National Cancer Institute 187, 198,
   204, 224
National Centers for Commun-
   icable Disease, Georgia 50
National Institute of Allergy and
   Infectious Diseases 202
National Institutes of Health 199,
   202, 210-211
National Tuberculosis Association
   80
NEOPLASTIC DISEASES 107
Netterberg, Robert 109
Newark Presbyterian Hospital 62
New York Academy of Medicine
   23
New York Academy of Sciences
   82
New York City Blood Center 201-
   202, 211
New York Medical College 19-20,
   34
NEW YORK DAILY NEWS 23
NEW YORK MICROSCOPICAL
   BULLETIN 60
NEW YORK NATIVE 192, 204,
   228
New York University Medical
   School 58
Nightingale, Florence 144

Nihmey, John 18
Nixon, Richard 198
Noguchi, Hideo 105
NORTHWEST MEDICINE 108
Nuzum, John 108
Nzaramba, Didace 209

O
Ollendorff, Ilse 169, 178, 181
ORANGE COUNTY REGISTER,
   209
Orgone Biophysical Research La-
   boratory 224
Ortleb, Charles 228

P
PASSION OF YOUTH 157
Pasteur Institute, Brussels 85
Pasteur Institute, Paris 205, 207
Pasteur, Louis 11, 13, 105, 116,
   125-131, 133-138, 144-145, 147-
   152, 166, 223
Paxman, Jeremy 194
PEBBLES ON THE HILL OF
   A SCIENTIST 81
Pillar, Charles 193, 213
Pink, Annie 160, 162
Pla Y Armengol, R 73
Plimmer, HG 106
Princeton University 61, 75
Priore, Antoine 224-225
PULSE OF THE PLANET 224

Q
QUEST FOR THE KILLERS
   210

R
RCA 79
Reagan, Ronald 207
Reich, Eva 160, 178, 181
Reich, Peter 169, 178, 181
Reich, Wilhelm 57, 152-153, 155-
   172, 175-183, 223-224, 272
Rhodes, Cornelius 79
Rife, Raymond Royal 224
Rosenthal, Lorraine 121-124, 156
Rowe, Lyon 97
Roy, Augustin 226

Russell, William 105-106, 248
Rutgers University 38, 50, 62

S

Schaumann, J 98
Schultz, Thomas 215
Scott, Michael 108-109
Seibert, Florence 80-82, 85, 93,
    104, 222, 272
SKIN AND ALLERGY NEWS
    206
Sloan-Kettering Institute for
    Cancer Research 86
Sloan-Kettering Memorial Hospital
    79
Smith, Lawrence W 62
Steinbrook, Robert 209
Stearn, AW 109
Stearn, AE 109
Strecker, Robert 190-191, 199
Sturdivant, BF 109
Sugrue, Tom 55
Swatek, Frank 40, 49
Sweany, HC 72
Szmuness, Wolf 201-203, 210-211

T

Taylor, Robert 109
Tedeschi, Guido 110
THE AIDS TIME BOMB 149
THE BION EXPERIMENTS 156,
    166-167
THE BLOOD AND ITS THIRD
    ANATOMIC ELEMENT 130,
    137-138, 143-144, 150
THE CANCER BIOPATHY 156
THE CANCER CONSPIRACY
    109
THE CONQUEST OF CANCER
    63
THE EVOLUTION OF LIFE 128
THE HEALING OF CANCER
    224
THE LAST EMPEROR (film)
    193
THE RIFE REPORT 224
THE SLEEPING PROPHET 55
THERE IS A RIVER 54

TIME (magazine) 78
TIME OF THEIR LIVES: THE
    DIONNE TRAGEDY 18

U

V

Veteran's Administration Hospital,
    Bronx NY, 31-32
Veteran's Administration Hospital,
    Long Beach CA, 33, 36, 47-49,
    51
von Brehmer, Wilhelm 109

W

Wayne State University, Detroit
    92, 222
West, John 149
Wilson, J Walter 40, 48
World Health Organization
    (WHO) 190, 199, 213-214, 216
Wuerthele, HH 58

X

Xalabarder, C 98-99

Y

Yale University 200
Yamamoto, Keith 193, 213
Young, James 107-108

About the Author

Alan Cantwell is a dermatologist and internationally-known scientific researcher in the field of cancer and AIDS microbiology. He is a graduate of New York Medical College, and studied dermatology at the Long Beach Veteran's Administration Hospital in Long Beach, California. Doctor Cantwell is the author of more than thirty published papers on cancer, AIDS, and other immunological diseases, which have appeared in leading national and international peer-reviewed medical journals. He is the author of the bestselling book, *AIDS: THE MYSTERY AND THE SOLUTION*, and *AIDS AND THE DOCTORS OF DEATH: AN INQUIRY INTO THE ORIGIN OF THE AIDS EPIDEMIC*. Born in New York City in 1934, Doctor Cantwell now lives in Los Angeles.

Aries Rising Press also offers:

AIDS: THE MYSTERY AND THE SOLUTION (Softcover, 210 pages, $9.95) by Alan Cantwell, Jr., M.D. — The most widely-acclaimed and informative book on AIDS and its relationship to cancer. Includes eight photographs of the cancer microbe in AIDS.

AIDS AND THE DOCTORS OF DEATH: AN INQUIRY INTO THE ORIGIN OF THE AIDS EPIDEMIC (Hardcover, 239 pages, $18.95) by Alan Cantwell, Jr., M.D. — A fully-documented account linking the AIDS outbreak in African blacks and American gays to biological experimentation with a new genetically engineered virus. A must-read book detailing the suppressed facts about AIDS.

Please make check or money order payable to Aries Rising Press, P.O. Box 29532, Los Angeles, CA 90029. Include $1.50 per book to cover cost of postage and shipping. California orders must include 6 1/2% sales tax. Allow 2-4 weeks for delivery.

CRITICAL PRAISE FOR...

AIDS: THE MYSTERY AND THE SOLUTION by
Alan Cantwell, Jr., MD

"Should be of great value to every physician, as well
as to everyone involved in protecting the health of
the community. Easy-to-read. . . contains the most
comprehensive world bibliography of work done by
trained physicians and technologists on AIDS, as well
as on a sadly neglected phase of cancer research."
  — **FLORENCE B. SEIBERT,**
  Ph.D., Sc.D., LL.D.,
  Emeritus Professor, University of Pennsylvania

"Well-written. . . should appeal to not only cancer and
AIDS researchers, microbiologists, and infectious
disease specialists, but also to the layman. A
fascinating, easy-to-read, informative, thought-
provoking book."
  — **DOROTHY BRANSON, Ph.D.,**
  Microbiologist, Columbus

"A daring and provocative book on AIDS. Doctor
Cantwell challenges established medical thinking
regarding the assumed viral cause of the AIDS
epidemic. As the mystery of AIDS unfolds in this
exciting book, the reader becomes appalled at the
indifference and unwillingness of the medical
establishment to consider an alternative infectious
cause of AIDS, and cancer as well. I urge everyone
interested in AIDS to read this remarkable book. . . it
will stimulate your thinking."
  — **ARMAND AUGER, M.D., Los Angeles**

AVAILABLE FROM LOCAL BOOKSELLERS OR
FROM ARIES RISING PRESS

CRITICAL PRAISE FOR...

AIDS AND THE DOCTORS OF DEATH by Alan Cantwell Jr., M.D.

The only book on AIDS the U.N. Health Officials DON'T want you to read!

"Who should read AIDS AND THE DOCTORS OF DEATH? Every man and woman on this planet!"
— **Wildfire Magazine**

"A provocative book that should cause more than a few waves of doubt in the troubled seas of AIDS research."
— **East-West Magazine**

"Riveting, I couldn't put it down."
— **Health and Healing Magazine**

"When Cantwell implicates agencies like the National Cancer Institute in a shadowy antigay conspiracy. . . his arguments deserve thoughtful consideration."
— **Wilson Library Bulletin**

"A well-written, entertaining book for those who love mysteries and conspiracies. . . not to mention. . . scientific matters."
— **Update Magazine**

AVAILABLE AT YOUR LOCAL BOOKSELLER OR THROUGH ARIES RISING PRESS